SUPERVISION AND
THE ANALYTIC ATTITUDE

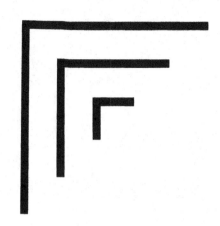

SUPERVISION AND THE ANALYTIC ATTITUDE

EDITED BY
CHRISTINE DRIVER MA
AND **EDWARD MARTIN** MA, MSc

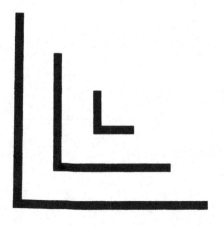

W
WHURR PUBLISHERS
LONDON AND PHILADELPHIA

© 2005 WHURR PUBLISHERS LTD

First published 2005
by Whurr Publishers Ltd
19b Compton Terrace
London N1 2UN England and
325 Chestnut Street, Philadelphia PA 19106 USA

British Library Cataloguing in Publication Data

A catalogue record for this book
is available from the British Library.

ISBN 1 86156 473 2

Typeset by Adrian McLaughlin, a@microguides.net

CONTENTS

CONTRIBUTORS

CLAIRE ALLPHIN is a Clinical Social Worker and Jungian Analyst in private practice in Oakland, California. She supervises interns at the clinic of the C. G. Jung Institute of San Francisco, at the California Institute for Clinical Social Work in Berkeley, California, and at The Psychotherapy Institute in Berkeley, California where she is also a founder of their Supervision Study Program.

RUTH BARNETT is a BCP and UKCP registered Psychoanalytic Psychotherapist and a member of BAPPS. Formerly a secondary-school teacher and currently involved in promoting Holocaust and genocide education, she approaches therapy and supervision with a learning model rather than a medical one. She has written several articles combining these professional interests.

STEPHEN CRAWFORD trained as a Psychodynamic Counsellor, a Psychoanalytic Psychotherapist and as a Supervisor at WPF Counselling and Psychotherapy. He is a member of the FPC, of BAPPS and is registered with UKCP. He works in private practice and also at WPF Counselling and Psychotherapy, where he is currently an Assistant Head of Training.

CHRISTINE DRIVER is a Professional Member of the SAP, a Training Therapist of FPC and a member of BAPPS. She is Programme Organizer, Seminar Leader and Supervisor on the MA/Postgraduate Diploma in Supervision at WPF Counselling and Psychotherapy, and teaches and supervises psychotherapists and counsellors. She has a private practice and is co-author and co-editor, with Edward Martin, of *Supervising Psychotherapy* (2002) London: Sage.

EDWARD MARTIN is a Professional Member of the SAP. He has organized, taught and supervised on supervision training programmes for WPF Counselling and Psychotherapy in London and within the United Kingdom and also for other professional bodies. He has contributed a number of chapters in professional books and, with Christine Driver, co-edited *Supervising Psychotherapy* (2002) London: Sage. He is in private practice.

ROSE STOCKWELL is a Psychoanalytic Psychotherapist and BACP accredited counsellor and supervisor. She is an Associate Member of the BAP, an Associate Professional Member of WMIP, a member of BAPPS and APP. She undertook the Maudsley Hospital Supervision and Consultative Course in 1988 and developed her supervision work in the NHS, voluntary sector and private practice.

MARY THOMAS originally trained as an artist and, subsequently, as a Psychodynamic Counsellor and Psychoanalytic Psychotherapist at WPF. She has worked for many years in Primary Care Counselling in the NHS. She is a Psychoanalytic Psychotherapy Member of FPC, working in private practice, and is a member of BAPPS. She supervises on the WPF Counselling and Psychotherapy Postgraduate Diploma in Psychodynamic Counselling and teaches and supervises on the Diploma in Supervision course for the same organization.

SANDRA THOMAS is a Psychotherapy member of The Hallam Institute of Psychotherapy and NWIDP, having originally trained as a marital counsellor with Relate and subsequently trained as a Psychoanalytic Psychotherapist, and then as a Psychoanalytic Supervisor.

MICHAEL WHAN qualified as an Analytical Psychologist with IGAP. He has published articles in a wide range of journals, including the *European Journal of Psychotherapy*, *Counselling and Health* and *The Psychotherapist*, and contributed chapters in two books: *Drawing the Soul: Schemas and Models in Psychoanalysis* (Burgoyne B (ed.) (2000) London: Karnac Books) and *Psychoanalysis and the Paranormal: Lands of Darkness* (Totton N (ed.) (2003) London: Karnac Books).

VERNON YORKE is a Professional Member of the SAP, and a Supervising and Training Therapist member of the LCP. He teaches and supervises for WPF Counselling and Psychotherapy and works in private practice.

PREFACE

Being a psychodynamic/psychoanalytic practitioner requires a working knowledge, and a depth of understanding, of unconscious processes and intrapsychic and interrelational dynamics. Being a supervisor, and supervising the work of others, requires the development of an array of skills, including the ability to discover, understand, translate and interpret unconscious processes and interrelational dynamics and apply this understanding within the supervisory relationship.

The genesis of this book evolved from ideas for research into supervision and the development of a supervision MA course. The aim was to consider the intertwining dynamics of supervision at depth, both at an intellectual and clinical level, and examine the way in which an analytic attitude and the use of analytic theory enables this.

The chapters of this book have emerged from this work and have been written from the perspective that a return to, and a rethinking of, basic psychoanalytic principles and an underlying analytic attitude are helpful in developing the skills needed for effective supervision work.

CHRISTINE DRIVER
EDWARD MARTIN
January 2005

FOREWORD

Supervision of analytic psychotherapy or counselling is a demanding business, and to write about it calls for impressive qualities of patience and observation. The sheer complexity of narrative involved in any case illustration is daunting: 'the therapist remembered the patient as having said . . . and having done . . . and herself as having said . . . and having done . . . and the supervisor chose to respond' to aspect 'x' of this complex communication, in the full awareness that it might only rather approximately relate to what actually occurred, in a consulting room, which, in all probability, the supervisor has never seen.

In these circumstances, the wonder sometimes is that supervision can be of any help at all. Moreover, in the British analytic world, there is a heroic tradition of refusing any technological help to gain a more concrete picture of what goes on in the consulting room, such as audio or video recording, on the grounds that this would foreground the externals of the situation and distract attention from the subtle interplay of phantasy and affect by which, so often, transference and countertransference can be recognised. What the supervisee remembers, how he or she presents it, usually several days later, to a supervisor to whom there will always be a further complicated deck of transferences, is held to convey or transmit the subtle interplay of conscious and unconscious communication more usefully than an external recording.

I use the word 'heroic' with a certain irony (there is room for research into the use of other methods of recording) but also with respect: it is indeed heroic to embrace a method that demands so much effort, especially of the supervisee, who is required to write long, always-inaccurate 'verbatim' accounts of sessions, for reasons that are so high-minded and intangible. This struggle to find a way to present clinical material perhaps illustrates the tension in psychoanalytic work of being both 'art' and 'science'. In supervision, too, the supervisor also has to work extremely hard to understand, internalize, conceptualize and interpret the material. This process is vividly demonstrated in the present book, edited by Christine Driver and Edward Martin. Christine Driver is a Psychoanalytic Psychotherapist and both she and Edward Martin are SAP Analysts.

One thing that strikes me particularly, when reading these chapters, is the careful attention their authors give to the interaction between supervisor and supervisee, and their belief that attention to this interaction can give rise to an understanding of what is taking place between the supervisee and the patient. In my own (older-generation) experiences of being supervised, the dynamics of the supervision itself were rarely if ever commented on. (I remember some rather stunningly overconfident supervision in consequence!) In this book, consideration is given to a more process-oriented approach; Christine Driver, in her chapter on language and interpretation, gives a nice example of how sensitively 'parallel process' can be worked with.

This new emphasis is healthy, in my view, at least up to a point. It is refreshing to see that there is a lively debate about it, rather than a consensus. Vernon Yorke addresses directly the sort of issue I have referred to above about the verbatim report of the session, which (in my view) is the fundamental 'material' with which supervision works. Yorke adapts Bion's theories, to do with analytic open-mindedness, and applies them directly to the practice of supervision. Supervisors should 'be without memory, desire and understanding', trust that the unknowable 'O' of supervision will enter with its 'invariants' undistorted into the reverie of the supervisor, and so on. Could such an approach risk overlooking the fact that supervision is task-oriented, that it is 'oversight' of something other than itself, namely therapy going on in another consulting room, and has a responsibility and a job-to-do quite distinct from therapy? It is a credit to Yorke's honesty that he ends with an example in which he felt his reverie distracted him from the central issues in the therapy.

Stephen Crawford, in a notably balanced chapter, examines these questions using a somewhat different analytic framework. (His references are mostly to psychoanalysts of the 'independent' group.) Crawford speaks of the 'limits to free association' in the supervisory situation and points out that the supervisor has many practical responsibilities to do with the patient's treatment, which need to be kept in view. He also notes that 'in supervision the supervisee is speaking of their work with the patient' – he or she is not free to merely free-associate.

Many other issues are brought up in these rich and varied discussions. Mary Thomas uses Winnicott's thoughts to make the important point that supervision needs to allow space for some freedom to 'play'. She reminds us that the transferences in supervision can be negative and stultifying as well as liberating and creative. Sandra Thomas writes about supervision in relation to training. Ruth Barnett strikes a very practical note in her comprehensive and useful chapter entitled 'Supervision: ethical practice and the law', in which she surveys the rapidly changing landscape of ethical and legal responsibilities of therapists. She provides a fascinating illustration of the overlapping but diverse professional dialects used by therapists, lawyers, doctors and ordinary members of the public, which can lead to subtle and sometimes gross failures of communication at times of great tension and worry. She comments also on such important issues as note-taking, confidentiality and the Data Protection Act.

Edward Martin writes perceptively on the important topic of the therapist's shame, one of the most powerful obstacles to remembering and honest reporting. He speaks of the way in which shame may inhibit the therapist's exposure of his or her work, particularly the countertransference feelings and phantasies that can be a crucial part of the communication of the session. It is an important part of the supervisor's job to be aware of the power of shame, and to avoid creating an atmosphere that enhances it. As Martin says, shame can also be powerful, and perhaps equally as inhibiting, when supervisors themselves are invited to expose their work in 'supervision of supervision'. My own experience of being in a supervisors' group parallels Martin's: the group found excellent reasons, session after session, to discuss general questions, or administrative or political questions, and to avoid the designated task of presenting our actual supervisory work for the scrutiny of colleagues.

I said that the wonder sometimes is that supervision can be of any help at all. In fact, good supervision can be profoundly helpful, at times even inspiring. In work with deeply disturbed, frightening or despair-inducing patients in the borderline or mildly autistic categories, supervision may be utterly essential to preserve the therapist's liveliness and capacity to keep thinking creatively.

There has clearly been a felt need in recent years for training in supervision, and the result is very interesting to someone of an older generation (such as myself) in which supervision was done by trained analysts or therapists simply on the strength of their initial analytic training and subsequent experience. A number of the contributors, including the two editors, have been connected with the pioneering training in supervision that was set up in 1985 by the London-based WPF Counselling and Psychotherapy.

It is of interest that this thoughtful book emerges from an organization with a pluralistic, non-dogmatic attitude to theory. While the overall tone of this book exemplifies the pluralistic approach, four chapters draw more specifically on the insight of particular analytic approaches. Clare Allphin returns to her roots when she applies Jung's alchemical model of the transference to the supervisory relationship; similarly Michael Whan takes his point of reference from Jung's work on typology. Balancing this is Rose Stockwell's chapter, written from the point of view of ego psychology, and Stephen Crawford's examination of free association.

This is not, therefore, a 'party book'. The references are wide-ranging and the questions debated transcend the traditional party lines. The reader will find that all the contributors write with a generous and humane tone, and it would surely be enriching to be supervised by any one of them. There is much in these chapters to challenge and develop the thinking of supervisors, would-be supervisors and supervisees from all points on the analytic spectrum.

DAVID BLACK
Member of the Institute of Psychoanalysis, London

Acknowledgements

The editors on behalf of themselves and the individual authors wish warmly to thank the following colleagues for their support, help, contributions and advice in the preparation of this book: Mary Banks, Richard Carvalho, Warren Colman, Elizabeth Driver, Lynsey Hotchkies, Jean Knox, Gertrud Mander, Jasmine Morton, Fiona Ross, Ineke van der Sanden and Eve Warin.

They would also like to thank their supervisees, who have trusted them with their work and from whom they have learnt so much.

The editors would also like to thank David Black for writing the foreword, Pastmos Verlag, Düsseldorf, for permission to publish the *Rosarium Philosophorum* pictures and Cambridge University Press for the two extracts from *Negotiating with the Dead: A Writer on Writing*, by Margaret Atwood 2002 (*Negotiating with the Dead*, © O.W. Toad Ltd. 2002).

ABBREVIATIONS

APP	The Association of Psychoanalytic Psychotherapists in the NHS
BACP	The British Association for Counselling and Psychotherapy
BAP	The British Association of Psychotherapists
BAPPS	The British Association of Psychoanalytic and Psychodynamic Supervision
BCP	The British Confederation of Psychotherapists
CPD	continuing professional development
FPC	The Foundation for Psychotherapy and Counselling
IGAP	The Independent Group of Analytical Psychologists
LCP	The London Centre for Psychotherapy
NHS	The National Health Service (UK)
NWIDP	The North-West Institute for Dynamic Psychotherapy
SAP	The Society of Analytical Psychology
UKCP	The United Kingdom Council for Psychotherapy
WMIP	The West Midlands Institute of Psychotherapy

A NOTE ON THE REFERENCES

Unless otherwise stated, 'SE' refers to the Standard Edition of *The Complete Psychological Works of Sigmund Freud* (volumes 1–23) translated by James Strachey and Anna Freud, assisted by Alex Strachey and Alan Tyson. London: Hogarth Press (1966). The various dates refer to the year of an individual paper's publication.

The Collected Works of CG Jung were edited by Sir Herbert Read, Michael Fordham and Gerhard Adler. London and New York: Routledge and Kegan Paul. The various dates refer to the year of an individual paper's original publication.

INTRODUCTION

SUPERVISION: THE INTERFACE OF THEORY AND PRACTICE

CHRISTINE DRIVER

Supervision has long been considered an essential part of clinical training and clinical work, and yet it occupies a place within the psychotherapeutic discipline that remains at the borders of theory and practice. Supervision is a discipline that is 'less than therapy and more than teaching' (Solnit 1970: 360), and this creates a tension that can leave supervisors in a place of uncertainty and has, perhaps, been partly the reason why supervision tended to become a more didactic discipline during the middle part of the twentieth century.

The growing awareness of the need for supervision to enable learning and understanding and to ensure ethical accountability in psychotherapeutic work has led to an intrinsic requirement for supervision within the profession. Supervision has therefore become established as a discipline of its own within the psychotherapeutic and counselling world, and the development of supervision trainings has promoted a consideration of the dynamics and processes involved. However, by and large, the supervisory world still retains a split between the theory that it engages with in relation to clinical work and the theory it engages with in relation to supervision. In some respects this puts supervision in a Cinderella position. Supervision is essential for the work, but it has, by and large, not felt able to put on the clothes and accoutrements of the profession that it works within because of the fear and anxiety that this will imply that it is therapy rather than supervision.

Supervision, however, stands at an interface between disciplines. Its task is to enable learning but not, necessarily, to teach directly. Its task is to enable internal shifts of perception and awareness in order to understand patients and their internal world and yet not become therapy. It incorporates, in Piaget's terms, both accommodative and assimilative learning (see Chapter 2's footnote: 19) as well as working with, and understanding, the dynamics of unconscious processes. It requires an understanding and awareness of the impact of organizational issues as well as requirements for assessment, ethical practice, clinical responsibility and the development of the clinical work with the patient. It is, in all senses, a multidimensional occupation which, like Ekstein and Wallerstein's (1972) concept of the Clinical Rhombus, Stewart's (2002) ideas about the Extended Clinical Rhombus or Perry's (2003) concept of the Matrix, has many different facets that interface with each other. Supervision is, therefore, a pluralistic and post-modern discipline which requires that it is informed by the theories, insights and understandings of related disciplines and, in particular, the discipline within which it occupies a core position and which it serves. In this case psychoanalytic and psychodynamic hypotheses and theories.

For centuries, writers, philosophers, alchemists, doctors, analysts, therapists etc. have formulated theories about the mind, psychic processes and the nature of the internal world in relation to the personality of the individual. From William James, Freud, Jung, Klein, Bion to Winnicott onwards, theories and hypotheses have been formulated in order to understand mental functioning, conscious and unconscious processes and the structuring and functioning of the internal world. These theories and ideas were developed in order to try to understand the mind and emotions of patients and to enable analysts, psychotherapists and counsellors, within the psychoanalytic and psychodynamic disciplines, to understand the internal world struggles of their patients and the intrapsychic and interpsychic processes that occur within and between people. In addition, theories about mutative processes and interpretation have been vital in illuminating the way in which understanding, meaning and internal shifts are generated. Just as these various theories have helped practitioners understand the dynamic processes inherent in the therapeutic relationship, they also provide ways of understanding the conscious and unconscious processes inherent in any relationship.

More recent studies into attachment theory (Bowlby 1981, Ainsworth et al. 1978, Holmes 2002, Fonagy 2001) and neuroscience (Schore 1994, Damasio 2000, Kaplan-Solms and Solms 2000) provide a further insight into the nature and development of mental and emotional functioning and the impact and influence of developmental, relational and intrinsic factors. These theories and discoveries provide a framework within which to understand individuals and the way they function internally and within relationships. Psychotherapeutic practice depends on such findings and ideas in order to make sense of the experience with the patient. It is vital for the psychotherapeutic practitioner to understand unconscious dynamics, such as transference and countertransference, projection and projective identification, and unconscious defences, in order to help bring to conscious consideration the internal struggles and relationship patterns that the patient is caught up in.

SUPERVISION AND THE ANALYTIC ATTITUDE

Supervision is a discipline that has a theoretical framework and body of theory of its own, but it is also enlivened and informed by the theories, insights and understandings of related disciplines. The purpose of this book is to consider some of the theories, ideas and formulations of related disciplines and explore how they further the development of supervision and the understanding of the personal in the interrelational work of the supervisory process. The supervisory process contains the interactive conscious and unconscious dynamics of patient, supervisee and supervisor and requires the supervisor to occupy a liminal space in order that experience and understanding are developed through awareness, reflection, thought and dialogue. The manner in which these phenomena are interpreted will, of necessity, differ from the therapeutic paradigm, but the processes through which they occur are the same. The challenge for the supervisor, in this liminal space, is to utilize the theoretical and conceptual ideas within the experience of the supervisory process in order to develop an understanding of the patient with the supervisee. The psychoanalytic and psychotherapeutic theories are our tools and monitors in a process in which an understanding of the impact and interrelationship of unconscious dynamics is vital.

Searles (1955) was one of the first to recognize how an understanding of the relational and unconscious processes in supervision is necessary in order to understand the dynamic processes that resonate within the supervisory dyad from the patient–therapist dyad. He examined the importance of utilizing countertransference within supervision and his conceptualization of the 'reflection process' was a key first step in unravelling the complexities and dynamics of the supervisory relationship. The significance of Searles' ideas was the way in which he used his understanding of unconscious processes, and the theories and hypotheses in relation to them, to consider the dynamics of the 'supervisor's emotional experience' (Searles 1955: 157–176) within supervision in order to understand the supervisory relationship and the patient. Searles' exploration of the reflection process, and Ekstein and Wallerstein's (1972) consideration of parallel processes, highlighted the fact that projective, transferential and unconscious processes were active within, and activated by, the supervisory arena.

To understand these phenomena, and to be able to interpret them in a manner in which understanding and insight is developed, the supervisor needs to bring their theoretical and clinical understanding to bear on the conscious and unconscious interrelationships within supervision. Frawley-O'Dea and Sarnat advocate that 'the process of supervision must be in some way analogous to the treatment approach advocated by the supervisor. In other words, the supervisory medium should convey the message the supervisor is trying to teach' (Frawley-O'Dea and Sarnat 2001: 3). In addition, the theories, models of the mind and interpersonal dynamics that we use in relation to the patient need to be used to understand the processes within supervision in order to parallel the medium and the message. This has been explored in Martindale et al. (1997), Langs (1994) and Driver and Martin (2002), but the aim of this book is primarily to consider theory in relation to supervision and how this informs our analytic attitude in terms of understanding the process, the relationship and our interventions and interpretations.

This book therefore explores how we can utilize the theories and understandings of the psychotherapeutic discipline to understand, develop and work within the process of supervision and the dynamic with the supervisee so as to develop our insight into and understanding of the patient. Clearly, within this the supervisor needs to be mindful of the ability and development of the supervisee. Some supervisees, new to clinical practice, may need nurturing towards a basic understanding of how to work with patients before they can progress to a more mindful place where they can examine and explore the patient's material with the supervisor. However, in any analytic and psychotherapeutic process, supervisor and supervisee need frameworks in order to conceptualize and verbalize experience. Theoretical constructs and models of the mind are the templates that provide such a framework and are the way in which supervisors and supervisees can make sense of the experience of the patient within the experience of supervision. Such an approach also allows the supervisor to utilize the triangular dynamic of supervision to enable the supervisee to gain an insight into the clinical work and the patient as well as modelling a process for the supervisee in terms of exploration, reflection, thought and understanding.

The application of theory to supervision therefore helps inform us, as supervisors, about the dynamics of the process and the dynamics of the interpersonal dimension of the supervisory relationship. The more we can understand what gets caught up into the supervisory relationship, the more we, as supervisors, can consider, understand and distinguish between the issues belonging to the patient, the learning needs of the supervisee and the interrelational processes and dynamics that need to be understood and worked with. Theories of the 'mind, health, pathology and treatment' (Frawley-O'Dea and Sarnat 2001: 2) have developed considerably over the past hundred or so years, but all revolve around the issue of trying to understand the internal world and the impact of, and relationship to, the external world. For a discipline such as supervision in which a consideration of the personal and interpersonal is involved, an understanding of psychological issues is vital.

The chapters therefore demonstrate the way in which theories and concepts are important tools and inform an analytic attitude in relation to the supervisory process. The authors explore a range of theoretical concepts that are not wedded to a particular school of thought but are rather the tools by which understanding has been developed and achieved. In the chapters the authors interweave key theoretical conceptualizations with clinical vignettes so as to bring the ideas to life and demonstrate the importance of their place within the supervisory paradigm.

The complex process of supervision involves integrity, understanding and awareness and requires a full understanding of 'the personal' in all its manifestations (cognitive, emotional, conscious, unconscious, psychological, physiological and ontological). What this book suggests is that an interdisciplinary approach to supervision and clinical work is essential in relation to pluralistic and post-modern thinking, understanding, conceptualizations and an analytic attitude. The key task of this book is to bring together the thinking and conceptualizations of the psychoanalytic and psychotherapeutic world so as to deepen understanding, reflection and the analytic attitude in relation to supervision and therapeutic processes.

REFERENCES

Ainsworth MDS, Blehar MC, Waters E et al. (1978) Patterns of Attachment: A Psychological Study of the Strange Situation. Hillsdale, NJ: Erlbaum.

Bowlby J (1981) Attachment and Loss: Volume 1. Attachment. Middlesex: Penguin Books.

Bowlby J (1981) Attachment and Loss: Volume 2. Separation. Middlesex: Penguin Books.

Bowlby J (1981) Attachment and Loss: Volume 3. Loss. Middlesex: Penguin Books.

Damasio A (2000) The Feeling of What Happens. London: William Heinemann.

Driver C, Martin E (eds) (2002) Supervising Psychotherapy. London: Sage Publications.

Ekstein R, Wallerstein RS (1972) The Teaching and Learning of Psychotherapy. Madison, CT: International Universities Press.

Fonagy P (2001) Attachment Theory and Psychoanalysis. New York: Other Press.

Frawley-O'Dea M, Sarnat JE (2001) The Supervisory Relationship. New York: Guilford Press.

Holmes J (2002) John Bowlby and Attachment Theory. East Sussex and New York: Brunner-Routledge.

Kaplan-Solms K, Solms M (2000) Clinical Studies in Neuro-Psychoanalysis. London: Karnac Books.

Langs R (1994) Doing Supervision and Being Supervised. London: Karnac Books.

Martindale B et al. (eds) (1997) Supervision and its Vicissitudes. London: Karnac Books.

Perry C (2003) 'Into the labyrinth: a developing approach to supervision'. In Wiener, J, Mizen R, Duckham J (eds), Supervising and Being Supervised. Basingstoke and New York: Palgrave Macmillan.

Schore AN (1994) Affect Regulation and the Origin of the Self. Hillsdale, NJ, and Hove, UK: Erlbaum.

Searles HF (1955) 'The informational value of the supervisor's emotional experiences'. In Searles HF (1986), Collected Papers on Schizophrenia and Related Subjects. London: Maresfield Library.

Solnit A (1970) Learning from psychoanalytic supervision. International Journal of Psycho-Analysis 51(3): 359–362.

Stewart J (2002) 'The container and the contained: supervision and its organizational context'. In Driver C, Martin E (eds), Supervising Psychotherapy. London: Sage Publications.

Szecsödy I (1997) '(How) is learning possible in supervision?' In Martindale B et al. (eds), Supervision and its Vicissitudes. London: Karnac Books.

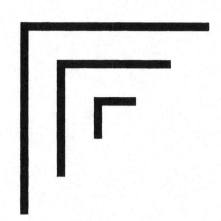

THE SUPERVISORY PROCESS

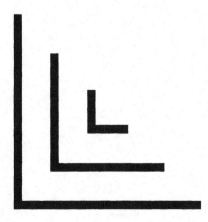

CHAPTER 1

THE UNCONSCIOUS IN SUPERVISION

EDWARD MARTIN

> *I see the moon, the moon sees me*
> *Under the leaves of the old oak tree.*
> *Please let the light that shines on me*
> *Shine on the one I love.*
>
> (Folk song)

INTRODUCTION

In 1899, the public first heard *Variations on an Original Theme*, the work of the composer Edward Elgar. These *Enigma Variations*, as they became known, are musical portraits of the composer's intimates and friends. While referring to them by initials superficially hid their identities, only a little detective work was required to reveal the names behind the initials. The real enigma refers to a melody other than the one heard at the outset. Despite much scholarly interest, that hidden melody has never been discovered, although it is a small frustration easily compensated for by the beautiful and masterly score.

The reader may feel uninterested, undermined, bemused or even hostile to my reference to music in a chapter on unconscious processes in supervision. However, this analogy highlights something very familiar to all therapists and supervisors. In therapy or supervision, the stated theme, the 'presenting problem', like the opening of this chapter, may be foreign or challenging, something that therapists and supervisors have to struggle to understand. The variations, often presented in the form of internal 'friends', form the content of subsequent sessions. While the presenting problem can be stated, what remains is the unconscious enigmatic theme that remains hidden. Entering this world and meeting these internal 'friends' is a privilege that rewards both sides of the supervisory encounter, an encounter whose objective is to discover the unconscious hidden theme.

As Elgar was composing, Freud was engaged in laying the foundations of psychoanalysis, which had, by 1915, developed into a sophisticated system of human mental functioning. This was the composition that Freud offered to the world, and from that many variations have been woven. This chapter revisits that theme again through the supervisory perspective, selectively choosing some of the variations that have emerged over the last hundred years

The unconscious is the *sine qua non* of psychodynamic psychotherapy. This alone justifies a return to the basic theories in a chapter on supervision, but, as Whan argues in chapter 12, theory is subjective. While the study of the theories of the unconscious forms part of all psychotherapy training programmes, every practitioner and every supervisor needs gradually to develop a personal theory of the unconscious that is usable, accessible and flexible enough to meet their own needs and those of their patients and supervisees. In chapter 5, Driver considers evidence suggesting that an individual's early environment influences the ability to 'relate to and understand the psychological characteristics of other people', in other words, the ability to form hypotheses about them. Yorke (chapter 3), using examples from fine art, reflects on how Bion's work provides a methodology that encourages creative work to happen in supervision. Matte-Blanco trenchantly states, 'I believe it is accurate to say that at the present moment a large proportion of analysts tend to avoid theorizing in order to concentrate . . . on clinical facts. Such an attitude seems ingenuous and those who adopt it seem to be unaware that in fact they are living on borrowed income' (Matte-Blanco 1975: 3). The challenge he throws down to the psychoanalytic community has reference to all involved in psychodynamic work. We either graft our hypotheses privately onto existing theories or, with sufficient courage (or secure enough attachment), develop a new strain of theory to enlarge the profession's repertoire and ability to respond to patients' material.

The intention of this chapter is to reiterate the original theme, a little augmented, on which supervisors will be able to construct their personal variations, their theory of the unconscious, whose true identity always remains enigmatic.

THE SYSTEM UNCONSCIOUS

Theories of the unconscious long pre-date Freud. Ellenberger (1970), in his classic work *The Discovery of the Unconscious*, reminds us, as does Whyte (1978: 4), that the 'discovery' of the unconscious mind was not a twentieth-century phenomenon. Macdiarmid, in a review of Ellenberger's work, describes that he painstakingly trawls through the researches of 'obscure doctors and practitioners one has never heard of finding 'what interesting things they observed and what good ideas they had about (the nature of the unconscious)', 'and how revealing when it is all put together' (Macdiarmid 1990: 135–139). Koestler, in his introduction to Whyte's (1978: unnumbered page) work, suggests rather unfairly that Freud gave the unconscious a 'clinical odour' and Jung gave it a 'mystical odour'. Unfair in that, while the awareness of the 'unconscious' mind had been well established before the *fin de siècle*, Koestler would appear to underestimate the revolutionary nature of Freud's work in establishing the dynamic nature of the unconscious. Whyte himself is more generous: 'Freud's greatness lies not in any of his particular ideas but in the fact that he compelled the race to face the problem of finding an adequate concept (understanding) of the unconscious mind. He showed, once and for all, (beyond any doubt) that the unconscious is so powerful that this task cannot be neglected' (Whyte 1978: 10, my parentheses).

Freud postulated that there were types of mental functioning that had their own laws, but which were fundamentally different from the thought processes that had been the object of traditional psychological observation. Freud called these 'primary processes' and demonstrated that they had specific characteristics in that they ignored categories of space and time, were archaic, derived from autoeroticism and sought to gain pleasure, night dreams being remnants of this archaic order. Additionally, primary-process images tended to fuse and readily replace and symbolize each other, both because there was a lack of organization and because each separate impulse sought independent satisfaction. So contradictions were completely inoperative, and opposite impulses, however extreme, flourished alongside each other. Freud categorized the unconscious (primary processes) as having the following features:

- condensation
- displacement
- timelessness
- absence of mutual contradiction
- replacement of external by internal reality   (Freud 1915: 187)

These Freud contrasted to what he termed secondary-process thinking. Secondary process was ego driven, thinking-related and adapted to the external world. It had an intimate connection with verbal reasoning and appeared to be subject to the laws of grammar and formal logic; it used bound rather than mobile energy and was governed by the reality principle, whereby un-pleasure of instinctual tension was reduced by adaptive behaviour. Whereas primary processes are exemplified by dreaming, secondary processes require conscious thought. Daydreaming and other creative activity involve a mixture of both.

Jung in his paper *Two Kinds of Thinking*, written in 1911, developed ideas along similar lines to Freud. Jung describes two types of mental processes, which he categorizes as two types of thinking: 'fantasy thinking' and 'directed thinking'. For Jung, fantasy thinking and directed thinking coexisted as two separate perspectives.

> *Anyone who observes himself attentively will find that the idioms of speech are very much to the point, for almost every day we see for ourselves, when falling asleep, how our fantasies get woven into our dreams, so between day dreaming and night dreaming there is not much difference. We have therefore two kinds of thinking: directed thinking or dreaming or fantasy thinking. The former operates with speech elements for the purpose of communicating, and is difficult and exhausting; the latter is effortless, working as it were spontaneously, with contents ready to hand and guided by unconscious motives. The one produces innovations and adoptions, copies reality, and tries to act on it; the other turns away from reality, sets free subjective tendencies, and, as regards to adoption, is unproductive.*   (Jung 1912/1967: para. 20)

Freud believed primary processes to be ontologically and phylogentically earlier than the secondary processes – hence the terminology. This suggests that he regarded the former merely as inherently maladaptive (Ryecroft 1972: 124). Jung adopts a different perspective, arguing that, while fantasy thinking was certainly characteristic of children and could be indicative of a certain type of pathology, it was not in itself pathological or infantile or maladaptive but the instinctive archaic basis of the mind that had grown collectively through the evolutionary process. Jung held for a more teleological view of the way in which humankind used this collective experience. Unlike a videotape on which the new overwrites the old, the new develops from the old incorporating the useful and usable. Jung's use of the word 'thinking' also strongly suggests that his view of the system unconscious was that it had its own structure, language and logic and acted as a counterbalance to the elevation of rationalism (Samuels et al. 1986: 47).

When patients undertake therapy, their problems are presented with a power and intensity that reflects their internal and unconscious conflicts and struggles. In the unconscious, conflicts, feelings and phantasies become symmetrically linked when A is treated as equal to B, and a disturbed or pathological state may be inferred when logically asymmetrical relations are treated as if they were symmetrical, because psychotic and unconscious thought processes tend towards symmetry. However, Freud and Jung were both formulating ideas about the nature of the unconscious and how it functioned in relation to ordinary human experience. The folk song quoted at the beginning of this chapter illustrates how the 'ordinary' psychosis of falling in love creates a symmetric logic that is not confined to human pathology but is part of 'ordinary' human expression and experience.

Matte-Blanco (1975: 12) augments and develops further the suggestion that the unconscious has a structure, logic and language. He asserts that Freud's work on the repressed unconscious has not been exploited to its fullest extent. He considers that Freud effectively abandoned the structural model by so slowly developing the concept after 1923 that its complete meaning and potentialities never fully came to light. 'We become aware that the idea of the unrepressed unconscious had fully *emerged* in Freud's mind during the last years of his life but it did not have time to arrive at a full development' (Matte-Blanco 1975: 78). Matte-Blanco finds that what he considers to be a 'disparate collection' (Freud's classifications) could be understood in terms of 'the interaction of a very few precisely defined fundamental processes, which can often produce highly complex dynamic mental structures' (Rayner 1995: 1). Using principles governing mathematical sets, and his own clinical experience, Matte-Blanco discovered that the apparent irrationality of his patients was not arbitrary but exhibited certain patterns, revealing an alternative or bizarre logic (Bomford 1999: 24). Matte-Blanco realized that primary processes exhibit bivalence: the absence of mutual contradiction and negation. From Freud's original classification, Matte-Blanco formulated two categories, symmetry and generalization, and it is these that will now be considered.

SYMMETRY IN SUPERVISION

This principle states that the unconscious treats the converse of any relation as identical with that relation. In the physical world, most relations are **asymmetrical**. An asymmetrical being is one whose converse is not identical to it.

Thus **asymmetrically**:

M is left of N	has the converse	N is right of M
M is before N	has the converse	N is after M
M is the mother of N	has the converse	N is the child of M

While **symmetrically**:

M is near N	has the converse	N is near M
M is the sibling of N	has the converse	N is the sibling of M

Asymmetrical relationships are the most commonly encountered. Most logical conscious reasoning and everyday thoughts about the physical world are conceived of asymmetrically; that is, relationships whose converses are not identical to them. Simultaneously, symmetrical relations will also be entertained in the mind, but they will remain consistently interwoven with logical thought providing an unspoken commentary that will not normally obliterate asymmetrical thinking. As an example, person A might begin to feel that they share much in common with person B. A might think, 'I am like B'; simultaneously, the thought might occur: 'I am the same as B.' This might increase a sense of warmth or closeness that would only become problematic if that second thought obliterated the asymmetrical reality that A is not B.

The principle of unconscious logic and symmetry has profound implications in the therapeutic endeavour. In order to function professionally and relate to the external world, the therapeutic relationship is conceived of as asymmetrical. Thus, a patient telephoning a therapist in distress is fine; the converse is not. However, unconscious logic conceives of the relationship as symmetric. Therefore, if patient X is in therapy with therapist Y, then therapist Y is in therapy with patient X. Jung (1972: 155–156) emphasizes the symmetry of the therapist–patient relationship, including the costs and benefits, not least the fact that both therapist and patient are changed by the end of a penetrating therapy. More pertinent for this chapter, however, is that, if X is the supervisor of Y, unconscious symmetric logic dictates that simultaneously Y is the supervisor of X – a dynamic exactly congruent to that described in therapeutic work.

This suggests that the nature of the supervisory relationship will depend as much on the way in which the unconscious of both supervisor and supervisee experience each other as on conscious or external factors, such as the relative experience or the seniority of the supervisor, the 'eminence' factor (Stimmel 1995: 609–618). In other words, it is the 'fit' that makes for a creative supervisory relationship. Much has been made of the necessity of ensuring that proper boundaries are observed, that is for example, boundaries between supervision and therapy, or between managerial supervision and clinical supervision. This applies both to situations in which supervisees choose their supervisors and to situations in which supervisees have their supervisors allocated to them. Always complicating matters and demanding consideration is the absent patient, completing the triangle.

The principle of symmetry also impinges on the setting and organization of supervision, and Langs' view of the setting and management of supervision is quite uncompromising (Langs 1994: 71–95). Supervision, he states, should be conducted identically to the way therapy is conducted, with strictly observed boundaries and the dialogue totally focused on the clinical work. This raises the issue of whether any advantage gained through peer learning in group supervision is outweighed by the disturbance caused by frame deviation, that is by a lack of symmetry. (See also Scanlon 2002: 219–235.) It also has implications for assessments of students (see chapter 9) and any organizational impingement that disturbs and distorts the frame.

The impact of unconscious processes in supervision in relation to the absent patient becomes realized, in part, through that extension of countertransference, the reflection process, whereby the relationship between patient and therapist is often reflected in the work between therapist and supervisor (Searles 1986: 157–177). The reflection process is an example of a symmetrical relationship, in that unconscious conflicts and anxieties become symmetrically linked within and between patient, therapist and supervisor in relation to the unconscious logic of each. This is illustrated in the following case.

A psychoanalytically trained female supervisee, in weekly supervision, presented time-limited clinical work from an agency. She introduced her patient, a senior and experienced nurse whose line manager had suggested that she self-refer to the agency following two major clinical errors in her work as a nurse specialist. The patient arrived stating she did not know what was the matter with her and that up to now her conduct and work record had been exemplary. She could not understand what had gone wrong. Gentle probing by the counsellor into the patient's background revealed a stable relationship, two achieving children and no financial worries or health problems. The patient appeared to be open and openly puzzled about her mistakes. By the end of the session, nothing had been found out and the patient left promising to return the following week. The supervisee was left feeling frustrated and a failure. Apart from that, her countertransference appeared blank, and she realized she had no strong feelings for the patient.

During the supervision session, the (male) supervisor observed that they (the supervisory couple) were both working hard to solve the puzzle – what could have caused this open, balanced, mature woman to make these two serious errors? The supervisee and supervisor found themselves agreeing that it was a mystery, that there seemed little affect in the consulting room or in the supervision room.

Both patient–supervisee and supervisee–supervisor are palpably stuck. Neither individually nor as a pair can they move. Both appear to be working hard at the material, both appear to evidence a good working alliance; yet nothing is happening. It would be surprising if all parties did not feel immense frustration but only one is conscious of it. Conscious, directed thinking appeared to colour the work. Allphin (chapter 7) uses one of a set of alchemical woodcuts that might accurately picture this scene: the king and queen (Figure 4) in the bath together. In the image, they appear together while being consciously unaware of any communication between them. Allphin writes, 'The discomfort or confusion may be thought of as information and unconscious communication from the patient and the therapeutic relationship that is being reflected and paralleled in the supervisory relationship.' There is an impasse in the supervisory encounter, and both supervisor and supervisee were stuck in a symmetrically linked place, which also reflected the stuck and blank place experienced by both therapist and patient. However, before discussing how this was resolved, Matte-Blanco's other concept, generalization, needs consideration.

THE PRINCIPLE OF GENERALIZATION IN SUPERVISION WORK

Matte-Blanco perceives that unconscious processes employ classificatory activities; they seek similarities between things. The unconscious therefore *does not relate to individuals but to classes* of which they are members. 'The system unconscious treats an individual thing (person, object, concept) as if it were a member or element of a set or class which contains other members; it treats this class as a subclass of a more general class, and this more general class as a subclass of a still more general class' (Rayner 1995: 22).

> *According to this principle the Unconscious, having first treated an individual as a class, tends to treat this class as the subclass of a more general class and so on to an unlimited extent. For example, an aggressive dog may first be registered as the class of all aggressive dogs . . . then as a subclass of all aggressive mammals, and that in turn as a subclass of all aggressive creatures of any kind.*   (Bomford 1999: 27–28)

Thus in the unconscious:

> *. . . an aggressive dog is felt to encompass the class of all dangerous aggressors – and thus perceived as presenting an infinite threat. The Unconscious having registered something as fearful or desirable registers it the same as other fearful or desirable things, in ever more inclusive circles. The individual who evokes a strong feeling thus potentially evokes this feeling to an infinite extent.*   (Bomford 1999: 27–28)

The disturbing intrusions of unconscious processes are present all the time in social as well as clinical settings. For example, while having a perfectly friendly conversation with an apparently reasonable stranger, a thought pops into one's mind: 'This person is a pig!' This of course might be true, and perhaps the unconscious insight might be worth heeding, even if social convention dictates that such thoughts are best kept with the thinker. When such disturbing images occur in the privacy of a consulting room, a different convention applies and a way needs to be found to express such thoughts appropriately, usually through an interpretation.

When a supervisor finds that a similar fantasy manifests itself within supervision, an appropriate response can be more problematic. Questions arise. How much is this a reflection process and how does the supervisor enable the supervisee to understand that that is where the patient's unconscious places him or her? How much is it an unresolved transference issue between supervisee and supervisor? How much is this part of the group process? Has this got institutional connections? Is it an indication of a requirement for further therapy (and how can that be enabled) or, as this transference has arisen within supervision, is it an indication of something that needs to be explored and understood within the supervisory framework? There are lots of possibilities requiring a wide range of responses.

To return to the case study:

> The discussion continued in a rather flat manner. Suddenly, the supervisor found himself totally gripped by a fantasy of getting out of his chair, reaching out to grab the supervisee's hand to pull her onto him. Associated with this was the certainty that that was what she wanted and passionate sex would follow. The strength of the fantasy was such that he felt the need to forcefully restrain himself from acting out.

This study reveals a number of issues about the nature of unconscious processes.

First, and needless to say, this is a **dangerous moment** in a supervisory relationship, and for this reason the relationship between supervisee and supervisor should be protected as securely as that between patient and therapist (Martin 2002: 121–132). This is a sort of reverie and according to Yorke in chapter 3 of this book, a 'preoccupying interlude', 'intensely personal' that may be considered 'embarrassing, shameful or 'psychopathological' and which would become 'psychopathological' if either acted out or repressed. It is a fantasy about the forbidden. Even if reciprocated, such a sexual embrace would be an embrace within the context of an imbalance of power.

The supervisor's fantasy focuses on a **symmetrical** relationship. The supervisor is certain that his passionate advances are wanted and will be welcomed. He fantasizes that he may take the supervisee's hand, they will fall into each other's arms, locked in a psychotic symmetric embrace. This is a fantasy about enchantment, Héloïse and Abelard, a fantasy that is about an urgency, sexual urgency, that would be reciprocated and result in passionate intercourse.

Rather than being acted on, the fantasy deserves to be understood. One way of understanding it is through the concept of **generalization** as a seduction or rape fantasy. In the therapy, both patient and supervisee express puzzlement, but it is the supervisee alone who was left with a feeling of frustration. The supervisee is holding an anxiety as to what it will take to get to the bottom of a problem whose symptoms relate to unconscious clinical errors. Perhaps the supervisor's fantasy is not so much about rape per se but the *generalized* characteristics of the rapist that are reflected in some aspect of the work. This may reflect an anxiety that there will be a rapine feeling in dealing with something sensitive in a time-limited framework. Although the therapist is female, unconsciously she may be conceived of as frighteningly phallic by the patient, who may fear being 'torn apart'. Equally, the patient may fear that it would be dangerous to allow herself to become vulnerable to this therapist in these conditions; perhaps representing an unconscious defence against her conscious wish to understand and resolve her difficulties.

Another way of considering this might be for the supervisor to reflect on the power of unconscious phantasy and the connection between this and the supervisor's powerful conscious fantasy. In other words, there might be a **symmetrical** *and* **generalized** link between patient, therapist and supervisor about fantasy/phantasy and an anxiety about their strength and power and the way in which they might induce 'clinical errors'.

The supervisor's task in this is to enable the work to progress and deepen, to enable his supervisee to find a way to engage in appropriate depth with her patient. The word 'appropriate' is important. Any interpretation has to keep in mind the possibility that the fantasy is not simply (and reassuringly) an example of the 'reflection process'; it also has to take into account the level of trust between supervisee and supervisor, the quality of their working alliance, the degree of sophistication of and the need to contain the supervisee. It would almost always be unwise to reveal the fantasy but only use it as a source of information for an intervention. However, the supervisor's task is to move this work on, and perhaps this could be begun by making a simple interpretation along the lines of 'I think that your patient is fearful of what may need to happen if she is to understand and resolve this matter in such a short time and you also may be unsure about how possible this is'.

Yorke (private communication) comments:

> *Depth can only come with confidence. Concomitantly confidence comes with depth. Encourage supervisees to get deep straight away, follow their reverie, feel free, let the theory come to them.* Not the other way round. *It is important that one works hard at difficult problems and finds ways through. This is what experience means. This is courage, not arrogance. The temptation as a supervisor is to become identified with a sort of trouble-shooter hero figure, sorting someone out of this or that difficulty or impasse with a borderline patient. This has something to do with the persona getting over-identified with the super-analyst image rather than a plain old supervisor one. Something may well get sorted out nearer the surface but whether it really gets to the rock bottom psychotic levels of impasse and symbol failure that is at the bottom of most difficulties is questionable.*

I understand Yorke to be criticizing an attitude towards supervision that severely limits working with unconscious processes, such as an overemphasis on technique, strategies and conscious knowledge, relating any difficulties to the supervisee's lack of such acquired knowledge. Institutional anxiety might, for example, result in a defensive use of supervision, policing the work rather than creatively working alongside the supervisees. This might take the form that clinical difficulties might be caused by the lack of consciously acquired skills rather than from unconscious defences in the supervisee–patient relationship.

THE WORDS TO SAY IT

The nature of the unconscious and its expression between patient, therapist and supervisor has many themes and variations, and the enigmatic nature of the unconscious attracts as powerfully today as it has throughout the history of the human race. Deep within the unconscious lies both the mystery of life and its meaning.

One of the aims of supervision is to enable the therapist to enable the patient to find words to express what cannot be expressed (or to discover feelings that pre-date words). This process is not about discovering anything new, anything not already known. The psychoanalyst Roger Money-Kyrle expresses this aim quite simply. It is 'to help the patient understand, and so overcome, emotional impediments to his discovering what he innately already knows'. He adds that 'all adult thinking, all later acts of recognition, are hampered by the difficulties which beset the first ones, and we all have some difficulties with these' (Money-Kyrle 1978: 443).

Money-Kyrle's statement beautifully and succinctly encapsulates Freud's great discovery and life's work, that of the dynamic unconscious. The 'unconscious' was the word used by Freud to describe both all that is not conscious in a given moment and the systems of the repressed contents unavailable to the pre-conscious-conscious system. Freud (1915/2001: 194) suggested early on the possibility that certain aspects of the unconscious contained phylogenetic elements. This suggestion was amplified both by Klein, who contributed her work on unconscious phantasy, and Jung, by insisting that the unconscious is primarily creative (and, incidentally, by adding the concept of the collective unconscious).

In 1931, Jung gave a lecture in Dresden that was later published as *The Practical Use of Dream Analysis* (Jung 1966). In this paper, he gives an example of his interpretation of a dream that makes disturbing reading that even in a Jungian training group gave rise to a certain degree of scepticism. It concerns a seemingly casual meeting between Jung and a colleague 'who always teased me about my dream analysis'. The colleague went on to say, 'I have had another idiotic dream' and told it. After some discussion Jung responded by warning his colleague not to go mountain climbing alone but to take two guides and follow them absolutely. This was laughingly dismissed by the colleague at the time but who, two months later, was buried under an avalanche but survived. Three months later, climbing again without guides, he was seen literally stepping out into the air while descending a rock face, killing himself and his friend (Jung 1966: 150–151). It can seem difficult to accept this account at face value for to do so would be to admit to the awesome power of the unconscious, but instead to try and explain or debunk it. It somehow doesn't quite fit in with a view of psychodynamics that seeks to bring the unconscious under conscious control and lends weight to Matte-Blanco's criticism of the profession for wanting to devalue the power of the unconscious.

> *In the course of its development psycho-analysis has become less psycho-analytic in the sense that, though it continues to deal with unconscious contents, it tends to treat them as though they were ruled by the same laws that are seen in consciousness and applied in the study of all other sciences.*   (Matte-Blanco 1975: 9)

Langs (1994: 1–2, 71–95) voices a similar criticism but from the perspective of supervision. He suggests that supervisors can use frame deviations as a way to avoid confronting the unconscious. His insistence that supervision should be conducted identically to the way therapy is conducted (regular time, privacy, attention only to the clinical material, no social exchange) is intended to enable the supervisee to enable the patient to encounter the deepest fears of personal annihilation that lie in the unconscious (Langs 1994: 25). Both Matte-Blanco's and Langs' criticisms need to be seriously considered by psychodynamic supervisors, for it is in that setting that supervisees will bring their own and their patient's fears, unconscious communications and defensive manoeuvres.

Matte-Blanco, while reminding the psychoanalytic community that the unconscious was and is the *sine qua non* of psychoanalytic and psychodynamic methodology, codified it. By doing so, he enabled the conscious mind to have a new approach to the system unconscious, and thus reawakened appreciation of the dynamic unconscious and of Freud's original genius. Anecdotally, newly trained therapists admit that the most challenging aspect of working with patients is working with the negative transference, the patient's resistance to knowing the 'facts of life', and with the bi-logic of unconscious processes personified particularly in countertransference experiences. This implies that supervisors need to find ways of responding to the patient's material in supervision so that through mirroring interpretations they can enable their supervisees to understand and grow in confidence of themselves making interpretative interventions appropriately. Often anxiety surrounds the use of part object language, or responding to the categorization of unconscious images. The task of finding the 'words to say it' – that is words that the patient can hear, digest and respond to – is one of the most fascinating tasks of supervision.

CONCLUSION

Like Elgar who left no clue to his hidden melody, the unconscious cannot be contained in any one theory; it will expand into them all and beyond. Confrontation with the unconscious will always have its dangers, and the conscious mind will always try and find escape routes. The art of the supervisor and the value of supervision lie not least in closing the escape routes and enabling the patient through the supervisee to find answers to 'overcome, emotional impediments to his discovering what he innately already knows' (Money-Kyrle 1978: 443).

Thus in the case study neither acting out nor a defensive retreat into techniques and strategies by the supervisor would enable the supervisee to address the patient's enigma, to begin to develop her own theory about her own unconscious and that of her patient's. Supervisee and supervisor would need to engage jointly on this task, a task that would gradually be tested by the patient's developing insight as well as against relevant published theory.

'Practical medicine is, and has always been, an art, and the same is true of practical analysis. True art is creation, and creation is beyond all theories. That is why I say to any beginner: learn your theories as well as you can, but put them aside when you touch the miracle of the living soul. Not theories but your own creative individuality must decide' (Jung 1928: 361 quoted in Beebe 2004: 178). For theory is the product of the conscious mind, but the unconscious is like Shakespeare's enigmatic midsummer night's fairy:

> Over hill, over dale
> Thorough bush, thorough brier,
> Over park, over pale,
> Thorough flood, thorough fire,
> I do wander everywhere,
> Swifter than the moone's sphere   (*A Midsummer Night's Dream* 1.1 1)

Something that cannot be contained within the realm of conscious thought.

REFERENCES

Beebe J (2004) Can there be a science of the symbolic? Journal of Analytical Psychology 49(2): 2.

Bomford R (1999) The Symmetry of God. London: Free Association Books.

Cross FL (ed.) (1957) The Oxford Dictionary of the Christian Church. London: Oxford University Press.

Ellenberger H (1970) The Discovery of the Unconscious. London: Basic Books.

Freud S (1909) Notes Upon a Case of Obsessional Neurosis. SE 10. London: Hogarth Press.

Freud S (1915) The Unconscious. SE 14. London: Hogarth Press.

Jung CG (1912/1967) Two Kinds of Thinking. Collected Works 5: 7–34. London: Routledge and Kegan Paul.

Jung CG (1966) The Practical Use of Dream Analysis in the Practice of Psychotherapy. Collected Works 16: 139–161. London: Routledge and Kegan Paul.

Jung CG (1972) Memories, Dreams, Reflections. London: Collins.

Langs R (1994) Doing Supervision and Being Supervised. London: Karnac Books.

Macdiarmid D (1990) A review of Ellenberger's work in 'Books Reconsidered'. British Journal of Psychiatry 156: 135–139.

Martin E (2002) 'Giving, taking, stealing: the ethics of supervision'. In Driver C, Martin E (eds), Supervising Psychotherapy. London: Sage Publications.

Matte-Blanco I (1975) The Unconscious as Infinite Sets. London: Duckworth.

Matte-Blanco I (1988) Thinking, Feeling, and Being. London: Routledge.

Money-Kyrle R (1978) 'The aim of psychoanalysis'. In Meltzer D, O'Shaughnessy F (eds), The Collected Papers of Roger Money-Kyrle. Perth: Clunie Press.

Rayner E (1995) Unconscious Logic. London: Routledge.

Ryecroft C (1972) A Critical Dictionary of Psychoanalysis. London: Penguin Books.

Samuels A, Shorter B, Plaut F (1986) A Critical Dictionary of Jungian Analysis. London: Routledge.

Scanlon C (2002) Group supervision of individual cases in the training of counsellors and psychotherapists: towards a group analytic model? British Journal of Psychotherapy 19(2): 219–235.

Searles HF (1986) Collected Papers on Schizophrenia and Related Subjects. London: Maresfield Library.

Stimmel B (1995) Resistance to awareness of the supervisor's transference with special reference to the parallel process. International Journal of Psycho-Analysis 76(6): 609–618.

Whyte LL (1978) The Unconscious Before Freud. London: Julian Friedmann.

CHAPTER 2

LANGUAGE AND INTERPRETATION IN SUPERVISION

CHRISTINE DRIVER

Language is a system of signs, different from the things signified, but able to suggest them.

(William James 1890/1950: 356)

INTRODUCTION

Words written in poetry, verse or story and words spoken in conversation, narrative and self-expression evoke and provoke thoughts, feelings, ideas and affects that stir the imagination, connect to memories and create meaning. Therapy, the talking cure, requires the use of words to describe, express, explore, understand and interpret the patient's narrative and experience. The therapist's ability to make interpretations relies on a number of factors, including an understanding of conscious and unconscious processes as well as an understanding of how words impact on and affect the other, the patient. How the therapist relates to and interprets to the patient is an important consideration in therapeutic practice. Of parallel importance is how the supervisor relates to the supervisee and interprets within the supervisory process.

Supervision is an important dimension of therapeutic work and acts as a forum in which clinical work can be spoken about, explored, understood, imagined and the work and understanding of the supervisee developed. Supervision impacts on the clinical process through the interactions of the supervisee and supervisor in terms of what is thought and said within supervision and the manner and style of the communication. The aim of interpretation within supervision is to engage the supervisee's internal world and stimulate dialogue between the conscious and unconscious in an internal dialectic that generates insight.

Studies on linguistics, learning, language, emotion and interpretation bring to clinical work a wealth of information and ideas about the interrelationship of communication and development. But, equally, they provide an insight into how the way we think about, and make conscious, what we are experiencing is affected by the language used and the style and manner in which we are spoken to. The issue of thought, language and communication, and their relationship to the conveyance of understanding, awareness and meaning within a relationship, is a vast area of study and research but one which is important within the parameters of the 'talking therapies'.

Any consideration of words, language and interpretation opens a rich palette that can provide detail as well as perspective. This chapter cannot hope to cover all the dimensions of this topic but aims to provide some ideas and considerations in relation to the subject of language and interpretation within the supervisory framework. This chapter explores three dimensions of this: the practice and process of supervision, the function of words and language and the issue of interpretation within supervision.

REFLECTIONS ON THE SUPERVISORY DIALOGUE

When a supervisor and supervisee meet to discuss a patient, their interactions take place at many levels. There may be a polite greeting and acknowledgement of the weather and a subliminal awareness of body language and emotional state. As the supervision session continues, and when discussing the presented session and the patient's material, the supervisor might explore the patient's issues with the supervisee in a variety of ways. The supervisor might give their associations and thoughts about the patient's material and link this to theory. They might engage in a dialogue or mutual exchange in order to enable the supervisee to link to the internal world of the patient and to make links that extend their understanding. In addition, the supervisor might make direct interpretations about the patient or interpretations about the process of engagement, between supervisor and supervisee, with the patient's material. Within supervision there are, therefore, a variety of dialogues, exchanges and mutual explorations.

The question that arises from this is: 'What is the aim of these interactive processes, dialogues and interpretations?' The aim within supervision must be to enable the supervisee to understand the patient more fully and to find meaning in the patient's narratives. This might require both supervisor and supervisee to make certain internal shifts to enable insight and a dynamic understanding of the patient and their internal world. The achievement, from time to time, of this dynamic understanding is crucial to the development of clinical work, but to enable this to occur requires the communication between supervisor and supervisee to touch on something that has the quality of linking emotion and thought in a way that transcends the original patterns of thinking and behaviour. The interactive processes and the words used therefore need to act within the internal world of the supervisee to create those 'aha' moments that shift understanding and assumptions. Piaget (1958)[1] makes a distinction similar to this when he talks about the difference between assimilative and accommodative learning. Assimilative learning refers to the gathering of new information, whereas accommodative learning requires a shift in our internal 'cognitive schemata' (Szecsödy 1997) and 'internal objects' (Martin 2002) to restructure previously held knowledge, and within therapeutic and supervisory processes it is accommodative learning which is of fundamental importance.

THE INNER AND OUTER EXPERIENCE OF WORDS

Our dialogues, and the way we gather 'this and that' (Meltzer 2003: 117), within supervisory presentations and exchanges all form part of the process of considering the patient's material and formulating hypotheses and interpretations. Communication within supervision is not just about language (Meltzer 2003: 285), but language and words make up the major part of the process, and any dialogue or interpretation requires the use of words. But what are we doing with language when we put things into words? Wittgenstein describes language as 'an instrument. Its concepts are instruments' and 'concepts lead us to make investigations; are the expression of our interest and direct our interest' (Wittgenstein 2001: 128: paras 569, 570). The importance of language in making connections and its use as an instrument is also pursued by Vygotsky in his explorations into the relation between words, language and thought. He comments that 'every thought tends to connect something with something else, to establish a relation between things' (Vygotsky 2002: 218). However, Vygotsky also goes on to say that 'thought is not begotten by thought; it is engendered by motivation, i.e., by our desires and needs, our interests and our emotions' (Vygotsky 2002: 254). The links between language and thought, and language, motivation and emotion are important considerations in relation to how we use speech and language because they hold the potential to convey both cognitive knowing and emotional understanding.

What we say, and how we say it, clearly influences the outcome of the communication in the listener, and in the case of the supervisee this is of vital

---

1 'Assimilative learning means that the new information is added to the previous, thereby increasing already existing knowledge. Accommodative learning means that encounters with new information result in a fundamental modification of existing cognitive schemata, so that the new encounter can be dealt with ... i.e. ... by restructuring previously held knowledge, points of view and theory' (Szecsödy 1997: 109)

importance in enabling and enhancing understanding. James recognizes the significance of words and meaning when he considers the way in which words can be used to generate static and dynamic meaning (James 1901: 265) and Ogden reflects on this when he cites James' comments that 'language fails to convey meaning (especially affective meaning) when it is used in a fashion that is focused on what it is saying as opposed to what it is doing' (Ogden 1999: 225). That is, we need to understand not only what an interpretation is saying but also what it is doing.

At whatever level of exchange the significance of what words 'do' is vital in terms of how they generate understanding and internal shifts within the other, in this case the supervisee. As Vygotsky also comments, 'Words and other signs are those means that direct our mental operations, control their course, and channel them toward the solution of the problem confronting us' (Vygotsky 2002: 106). Language and words, therefore, have many functions within the supervisory process and have many attributes. They describe, define, categorize, appraise, explore, reflect, create meaning, generate emotion and touch the internal world and internal objects of the listener. Within each of these attributes there can be nuances of meaning in relation to the tone of voice, manner and type of associations, critical and evaluative references, and empathic and discerning understanding. Words also take the listener somewhere else. Words are nouns, verbs and adverbs. They name, act or describe; they link, connect and move; they possess both cognitive and emotional impact; words 'do' as well as 'say' and take the listener on a journey that engages external and internal dialogues.

This may all seem too specific in relation to the encounter with the unknown within supervision. The supervisee might bring an extensive narrative about the session or talk freely, but, by and large, the supervisor does not know what to expect when the supervisee arrives for supervision. This presents the supervisor with a challenge in terms of how to engage with the material and with the supervisee. Comments and interpretations may deaden or surprise, but they may also generate cognitive understanding and link to emotional understanding in a way that shifts 'internal objects' (Martin 2002) and enable integration. It is this process that is part of the complex activity of creating understanding and the finding of meaning. Interpretation in therapeutic work has been written about extensively, but of equal importance is the issue of interpretation within supervision. Words, and what they do in interpretations, comments and reflections, contain the potential to connect thought and emotion and link to integrational processes that contain within them the possibility of creating understanding and generating meaning within both supervisor and supervisee and ultimately the patient.

REFLECTIONS ON INTERPRETATION

One of the first key papers to consider the issue of interpretation in therapeutic work was that by Strachey (1934). He makes the distinction between transference and extra transference interpretations and emphasizes the importance of transference interpretations in holding a key position in therapeutic work and mutative experience. Strachey describes mutative transference interpretations in terms of bringing to consciousness a 'small quantity of the patient's id energy' (Strachey 1934: 142), when it is 'alive and present', and in this way the 'patient must experience something actual' (Strachey 1934: 150). It would seem therefore that, for Strachey, mutative transference interpretations speak to the immediacy of affect emerging from the patient when it is alive in the session. However, what is also important to consider is the impact of the language and dialogue between therapist and patient, and supervisor and supervisee and the potential richness of any therapeutic encounter in terms of where language and dialogue take the participants. In other words, what words 'do'.

Since Strachey's seminal paper, many writers have explored and expanded the subject of interpretation. Winnicott (1980), in *Playing and Reality*, considers that one important aspect of interpretation is to allow the patient to see the limits of the therapist's understanding, which will allow the patient to work towards their own understanding. Fordham proposes that interpretations could be considered as being an 'intellectual act', a means of making a connection or be affect based and transference related (Fordham 1986: 113) and that 'if the aim of interpretations is to expand consciousness, they are synthetic' (Fordham 1986: 117), in that the aim is to provide meaning and understanding for the patient. Bollas speaks of the use of interpretation to 'structure experience' (Bollas 1991a: 21) in relation to the 'aesthetics of the transformational-object situation' (Bollas 1993: 48). Casement (1999) considers the importance of providing 'fresh insight' rather than cliché, and Ogden reflects on how 'the analytic experience is a fabric woven from the warp and woof of aliveness and deadness, of reverie and interpretation, of privacy and communication, of individuality and intersubjectivity, of the seemingly ordinary and deeply personal, of a freedom to experiment and a groundedness in existing forms, of a love of imaginative language for itself and the use of language as a means to a therapeutic end' (Ogden 1999: 19).

Understanding the way that dialogue and interpretation impact on and affect the supervisee and patient and their inner objects is fundamental to psychotherapeutic technique and vital within supervision if it is to be a therapeutic relationship in the service of the patient. To consider the issues concerning interpretation in the supervisory relationship it is useful to build and expand on the conceptualizations of interpretations within the therapeutic relationship.

However, this raises interesting questions in relation to interpretation within the multidimensional experience of supervision because the aim of the supervisory process is to develop insight, awareness and understanding within the supervisee about another, the patient.

INTERPRETATION IN SUPERVISION

Interpretations within supervision have many functions. These include reflections in relation to the patient's inner world, considerations of the patient–therapist interaction, use of the supervisor's countertransference to interpret the reflection process, interpretation of the dynamic of the triangular transference and the imparting of information and theory. Supervision can be a one-person, two-person and three-person dynamic, and a consideration of the material presented and the interactions and dynamics of the patient–therapist–supervisor triangle need to reflect that. The following example considers these dimensions and the importance of understanding the dynamics within the supervisory relationship in terms of where an interpretation is placed and what it is doing.

> A supervisee presented a patient who had spent the session describing the complexities of her family and her struggle in relation to her parents and siblings at a recent wedding. The supervisor, in considering the material presented by the supervisee, struggled to make sense of what the supervisee was presenting in relation to the patient's issues as well as the supervisee's concerns. In order to try to generate understanding the supervisor commented, somewhat simplistically, to the supervisee, 'This material, that the patient is presenting, is all about Oedipal struggles.' In response, the supervisee commented, 'Well, yes. I suppose it is.' The interchange enabled a thought to be communicated and, theoretically, this interpretation was correct, but its didactic, one-person nature did not develop understanding by the supervisee, or affect internal processes.

Interpretation in supervision, just as in therapeutic processes, needs to engage the supervisee in the processes of thought, imagination, association, conscious awareness of affective and unconscious processes plus many other internal and dialectic processes that engage both subjective and objective experience. Ogden makes the very pertinent comment when he reflects on 'the stifling effect on imagination of our efforts to define' (Ogden 1999: 3). Supervision therefore sits within a paradox. On the one hand, the content and processes are needing to be defined in order that their specific meaning is identified and made conscious; on the other hand, the internal processes within and between supervisor and supervisee need to be opened out to allow both parties to explore, imagine, think and find a new perspective and new understanding of the patient, and their internal world, so that the meaning for the patient, and the patient in relation to the therapist, is discovered.

> Following on from the above interchange, the supervisor reflected on the outcome of her interpretation and realized that her comment had been absorbed by the supervisee as a fact which did not generate further thought or reflection. The supervisor then made an interpretation to the supervisee on what was going on between them in relation to the supervisory process. She commented, 'I feel my previous comment has created something dead in this process which can't go anywhere.' The supervisee replied, 'Well, I understand what you mean by the patient being caught in an Oedipal struggle, but I don't know what to do with that, it sort of feels: "Well, so what?" because I don't know how to use that with the patient; she just feels angry about being left out.' This second interchange with the supervisor moved the supervisory dialogue from a one-person didactic comment to a two-person dialogue between supervisor and supervisee in which the more personal content of the patient and the patient–therapist interaction could emerge. Within this more exploratory form of language, and the manner in which the feel of the interrelational process was put into words by the supervisor, both supervisor and supervisee could have a space for reflection about the patient and the dynamic of the interaction between the patient and the therapist.

This latter interchange between supervisor and supervisee developed into a two-person interchange about the third, the patient. The interpretation that the supervisor used opened out a consideration of the dynamics of the process in relation to the content and the possible parallel dynamics, and this enabled space to engage the supervisee in self-reflection and internal dialogue. This dialogue also enabled the supervisee to speak about the relationship with the supervisor, and this seemed to free up the interaction between them, enabling a space for thinking and reflecting.

This process is of primary importance in supervision and underpins an important dynamic that makes supervision so essential. It also reflects the understanding that Vygotsky (2002) brings to the function of speech and communication in which he proposes that the primary function of speech is that it allows the development of dialogue, communication, egocentric speech and subsequently inner speech. In some ways this parallels the formulations made by Casement (1985) about the manner in which the external supervisor is internalized and eventually becomes the internal supervisor and part of the professional self of the practising therapist. What Vygotsky's work, and that of others, conceptualizes is how language and communication is part of the developmental process of internalization through the development of 'inner speech' (Vygotsky 2002: 34).

The purpose of supervision, in terms of the dialogue about the patient, is to enable the supervisee to conceptualize and understand the inner world of the patient, and the various transference and countertransference dynamics, in order to bring mutative understanding to the work with the patient. To enable the supervisee to conceptualize this, thoughts, words and structure need to be brought to bear on the content and experience of the work. As Vygotsky comments, 'it is *the* functional use of the word, or any other sign, as *a* means of focusing one's attention, selecting distinctive features and analyzing and synthesizing them, that plays such a central role in concept formation' (Vygotsky 2002: 106). In addition, however, the words that are spoken, and the interpretations that are made, need to engage the internal world of the supervisee in order that they have true meaning and generate an internal shift which allows for a conscious awareness of the issues that the patient and therapist are struggling with.

> The supervisor, in the example, began to consider the interchange that she and the supervisee were having about the patient and realized that the dynamic generated by the patient, the session's content, and the contents of the supervision and the supervisory relationship could not maintain a focus on all three participants in the dynamic and that this tended to happen whenever this particular patient was being presented. The supervisor, reflecting on this, realized that her interpretations had not included the three-person dynamic of the triangular transference inherent in supervision. Through a consideration of the issues involved, she made the following interpretation to the supervisee. 'It seems to me that we tend to talk about the patient so that she gets left out. This seems to be what the patient describes, as though no one really wants to know what she thinks and feels, and so she struggles with feeling lost, ignored and misunderstood, perhaps just as you don't know what to do when I make my comments and you feel left out by my thinking.'
>
> This complex interpretation endeavoured to encapsulate the triangular dynamic inherent within the supervisory relationship and offered the supervisee a range of patient-related areas to explore. The supervisor was unsure at this point whether the supervisee was ready for such an interpretation but allowed the subsequent silence in order to give the

supervisee time to internalize, digest and have her own internal dialogue about the issues and dynamics involved for the patient. After a few minutes, the supervisee commented, 'I think when I present this patient I present the confusion about her struggle because I am frightened to think about what she really brings. It's easier to have your thoughts, and I think the patient does the same thing. It's easier for her to have my thoughts, or at least my comments, because I think she is frightened of what she might think and feel in relation to her situation.' The supervisor commented, 'What do you feel she is frightened of?' After a pause, the supervisee replied, 'I think she is frightened to think about how needy and dependent she is on others and on me and yet she creates that dependency, and that's sort of what I do here too.' The supervisor responded, 'So what you're saying is that the patient brings a fear and a desire about dependency and doesn't know how to express it but hopes that others will do it for her?' The supervisee replied, 'Well, yes. I think that's right. I think she longs for others to recognize what she fears; she wants others to think for her, to say it for her.'

The importance of this latter dialogue is that the interpretation by the supervisor, based on the triangular dynamic, enabled a reflective space in which both supervisor and supervisee could explore. To some degree the development of understanding by the supervisee, within this triangular dynamic of the reflection process, depended on the developmental level of the supervisee. A supervisee new to clinical work may not have the capacity to internalize, twin-track and reflect on the simultaneous input of the patient's material and the supervisor's interpretation and may need a more directive exploration. However, the supervisor needs to mirror a 'reflective function' (Fonagy 2001; Driver, chapter 5) for the supervisee and, in addition, generate reflective interpretations that speak to the affect and dynamic of the triangular transference in order to enable the supervisee to understand the unconscious issues and internal objects of the patient.

One of the many functions of the supervisory process therefore is to stimulate thought and reflection on the material presented by the patient in order to generate a meaningful understanding of the patient's internal world, internal conflicts and how they affect the patient's outer relationships. When a supervisee presents the content of a session or sessions with a patient, and perhaps their associations to it, they are putting into words the patient's thoughts and feelings through the medium of their own. Not only does this have unconscious reverberations, as Searles (1955) identifies, but it also has implications in relation to the language used and the thought processes that the language accommodates and connects to. In the interchange in each of the supervisory examples above, the words were doing and saying different things. In the first, the interpretation defined but remained static; it did not lead the supervisee anywhere but did provide a thought, an idea and perhaps a concept on which other thoughts could coalesce. In the second and third examples, the interpretations were more dynamic; the words were inclusive of the process, reflected on the dynamic and opened out the experience. They made connections between thought and emotion and took the supervisee to a place where they could find new insight in relation to the patient.

A further dynamic within supervision is the interrelationship between supervision and the therapy and the therapy and the supervision. An understanding and interpretation of this dynamic may also bring insight into the patient's inner world, as the following example identifies.

> A supervisee saw a patient three times a week for therapy and came for supervision weekly. It became apparent that her interpretations and relationship to her patient, when the supervision and the patient's session were on the same day, were intrinsically different to the way she related to her patient six days on from supervision. In the patient's session, which occurred later on the same day as the supervision, the therapist made empathic reflections and interpreted psychodynamically in relation to the patient's emotional and 'baby' needs. When the therapist reported the sessions six days on from the supervision, she commented that she felt that the patient was often rivalrous with her and that she felt she had to work hard to find her own internal supervisor. In considering the flow of the sessions over the weeks, the supervisor commented that it seemed as though in the session following the supervision the supervisee could take support from supervision and that this enabled a sense of an internal couple that could contain, hold and understand the patient. However, in the sessions six days on it felt as though the supervisee had to find her own internal supervisor and that she felt more like a single mother. In the light of the patient's history and material, it was then possible for supervisor and supervisee to explore the impact of the patient's experience of a father who was often not present and a mother who had to frequently cope on her own and where the children became rivals in relation to the mother's needs.

Interpretation in supervision can therefore speak to, and contain, the various dynamics of the work in relation to the patient's material. Interpretation can speak to the broader dynamic as well as to the supervisor–supervisee relationship, but it can also speak to the embodied experience of the impact of the patient's material.

LANGUAGE: EMBODIED AND SYMBOLIC

Narrative, within the therapeutic encounter, embodies all aspects of the self. Communication via unconscious processes, projection, projective identification, transference and countertransference can convey experience at a physical level as well as at an emotional or cognitive level. Julia Kristeva categorizes words and language in relation to the signifier and the signified (Moi 1986: 25) and makes an important distinction between the semiotic (bodily experience) and the symbolic. For Kristeva the semiotic is a pre-Oedipal language expressing visceral, emotional and body texts in relation to the physical experience of the infant with the mother (Jonte-Pace 1997: 244). In contrast, the symbolic is the 'space of language, culture, morality and society' (Jonte-Pace 1997: 244) and links much more to the language of the Oedipal and post-Oedipal and the influence of separation, culture and the father.

In supervision, language may tend towards the 'symbolic order' in that it focuses on the accepted 'cultural and linguistic meanings' (Jonte-Pace 1997: 244); however, for Kristeva, the symbolic is 'constantly disrupted by the semiotic' (Jonte-Pace 1997: 244). Not only is the semiotic pre-Oedipal and pre-linguistic; it is 'initially structured and directed in relation to the mother's body', whereas the symbolic order is of 'a patriarchal social order' (Jonte-Pace 1997: 244). The importance of Kristeva's explorations is that they contain a consideration of the significance of the dialectic between at least two domains of expression and experience, a dialectic that may occur between the pre-Oedipal and the Oedipal, the semiotic and the symbolic, the body and the mind, the artistic musicality of expression and the social and cultural embodiments of thought.

Within supervision it is perhaps all too easy to fall into, or be pushed into, being the verbalizer of the social and cultural embodiments of thought in relation to theories, dogmas and ethics (for a discussion on the subjectivity of theory see Michael Whan, chapter 12). Interpretations that just remain at this level remain static, much as Casement describes in 'Interpretation, Fresh Insight or Cliché' (Casement 1999, Chapter 2). Experience of projective identification and the transference tells us, however, that the intrusion of the semiotic, the visceral, bodily experiences, are part and parcel of therapeutic work and emerge within the processes that become paralleled in supervision. Internal consideration of these visceral, bodily dynamics is important for the supervisor and needs to play a part in the interpretation of the clinical material in terms of the underlying tones of affect and the form the experience takes. As Siegel comments, 'our internal experience of emotion becomes in essence the "music of the mind"' (Siegel 1998: 7). The way that this might be interpreted in supervision will vary. The mode of interpreting directly to the physical level of experience does, in some sense, speak to the semiotic, but this denies the developmental status of the supervisee as being someone who also operates within and from the symbolic. Interpretation within supervision therefore needs to find a way to speak to, and relate to, both from time to time.

> An illustration of this occurred when a supervisee, new to clinical work, presented her patient. She spoke quickly and frantically about all the patient had told her and described the onslaught she had experienced from the patient. The supervisor felt overwhelmed by the input and somewhat sick and dizzy. She then interpreted quite directly from her experience with the supervisee and commented, 'This is overwhelming. It's just like there's shit everywhere and nothing can be held inside.' This direct reference to the physical, preverbal level of experience then enabled both supervisee and supervisor to consider the nature of the patient's early maternal relationship.

Words and language therefore have many functions within the therapeutic and supervisory relationship, and, although it is important not to become self-consciously stuck by trying to find the (supposedly) right words, it is also important to consider the words that are used, and the way they are used. The use of metaphor (as in the above example) and symbol enable exploration of a broader perspective that can take the listener to a different place in their aware-ness and understanding. Reflections on what we say and how we say it help in understanding the processes we are caught in. Simultaneously, it is important to be aware of the language we use so as to consider what words 'say', what words 'do' and where they are directed.

INTERPRETATION AND THE IMPORTANCE OF UNCERTAINTY

One of the dangers in writing about the nature, function and purpose of inter-pretation is of falling into the trap of sounding dogmatic and didactic as though interpretations can be formulaically defined. Casement points out that when interpretations become formulaic and cliché-ridden they 'promote an intellec-tualization of the analytic experience' and cease to provide 'fresh insight' (Casement 1999: 17). Learning by rote has long been considered antithetical to true learning and understanding. A learning culture needs to create an active engagement in a process in which there is reflection, thought and observation through which understanding and insight develop. This is certainly necessary in supervision, and Mander comments, 'objectivity, sustained observation and clear-headedness (not to be confused with intellectualization or cleverness) are necessary qualities of the good supervisor' (Mander 1998: 59); equally, these are also the qualities that supervisors are endeavouring to nurture within their supervisees. Although didactic comments may sometimes be necessary, on their own they stifle thought and independent reflection by the supervisee. When interpretations continually speak from certainty, they deny an engagement with the other by the other. An interpretation needs to create movement within the listener so that they can meet and engage with the process and the experience. The paradox is, therefore, that, although the aim of an interpretation is to provide meaning and understanding, it requires a degree of uncertainty to enable movement, thought and emotion within the listener.

We 'need uncertainty to create knowledge' (Davies 2003), a comment attributed to Heisenberg's ideas about the significance of uncertainty in relation to the properties of matter in an exploration of his work. Heisenberg considers that 'there is a limit to the precision with which the position and the momentum of an object can be measured' and that 'the more precisely one of the quantities is measured, the less precisely the other is known' (Heisenberg 2001: 1). These relational ideas about the properties of matter and uncertainty could equally well be attributed to the properties of thought and the medium of thinking, awareness, internal processes and formulations and interpretations within either the therapeutic or supervisory encounter. Heisenberg's principles would indicate that as soon as we comment on, or interpret, the experience of the relationship the relationship changes and the focus shifts and that the more one perception is defined so the less precisely the other (the dynamic meaning) is known or understood by the other. This reflects an important consideration regarding interpretations within the therapeutic and supervisory relationship. If the supervisor defines too much, the supervisee is prevented from relating to and interacting with the experience. As Gee comments, the supervisory process needs to be 'relating, then defining' (Gee 1998: 9).

Relating and uncertainty are present in any interactive process in which external interactions affect and influence internal objects and internal processes, and it is through the processes of inner speech, reverie, imagination, reflection and thought that understanding and meaning are developed. It is also important to view any interaction from a tangent so as to perceive the direction of the interpretation as well as what it moves away from, that is to consider what the interpretation contains and what it excludes because what it excludes might also contain important information.

An example of this occurred when a supervisor was able to reflect that he was always making comments and interpretations directly about the patient within a one-person dynamic and excluded the supervisee from the considerations. He was able to use his understanding to interpret this for the supervisee in terms of how the patient's material drew him to just considering the patient and that maybe the patient could only tolerate a one-person and narcissistic relationship. This reflection by the supervisor, from the use of his objective reflections on his countertransference and manner of relating, gave the supervisee an insight into a dynamic that might be generated by the patient. The supervisor's reflection therefore presented the supervisee with a concept in relation to the experience, which enabled a broader understanding of the patient.

The importance of uncertainty and limitations is also explored by Winnicott. He focuses on interpretation in terms of there being an expression of the limits of knowledge and understanding, which allow the patient to play and to find their own answers (Winnicott 1980: 102). In addition, Casement speaks of the seductiveness of certainty and that if 'too much weight is given to what is known the unknown remains elusive' (Casement 1999: 4). Bollas considers that interpretations 'are appreciated less for their content, and more for their function as structuring experience' (Bollas 1991a: 21). He goes on to make the comment that 'the analytical process . . . involves transforming facts into reflected objects, into mental objects, that in turn link up with other mental objects, to become part of intersecting chains of signification enriching a person's symbolic life, and also constructing a mental structure that can enhance the individual's mental processing of the facts of his existence' (Bollas 1991b: 68). From this, Bollas considers that, for an interpretation or comment to be insightful and promote insight, 'it must undergo a topographic return: from the analyst's comment to a preconscious holding area (an inner mental space) where it evokes instinctual representations, unconscious affects, and unconscious memories, and then returns to consciousness after some inner work has occurred. An analytic idea, then, has been transferred into an insight because what was only a theory now bears the patient's instinctual, affective and memorial print' (Bollas 1991b: 96).

Bollas' ideas are relevant in relation to supervision because, although the process in relation to the patient's internal world is once removed, we, as supervisors, need to evoke the same mental processes within our supervisees. That is, the supervisor's comments and interpretations need to engage the supervisee's 'inner mental space' so that the inner work of conscious and unconscious connections occurs within the supervisee. This then enables the supervisee to make internal links and gain insight into the patient, and the patient's experience, in a manner that has personal meaning to the supervisee and subsequently the patient. Verification of the process comes through encoded communications (Langs 1994) or conscious insight by the patient.

CONCLUSION

The purpose of interpretation in supervision is to offer a formulation to the supervisee that enables them to gain insight about the patient. The nature of this process is via the interaction of words, language and interpretations, but it is also within the fluid function of 'not knowing', reverie, listening and silent contemplation and the way that interactive processes enable and develop reflection, insight and awareness. Key to this consideration is the issue of what interpretations do and that 'they are most helpful when they engage the supervisee's inner world and promote an atmosphere of thoughtful reflection within the supervision session' (Colman 2004, personal communication). Words, language and communication are the ways in which we try to express and understand the experience and pain of the patient and give signposts that connect to their meaning. Within supervision, interpretation is not only about gaining insight but also about the development of the supervisee's understanding and ability to work professionally and ethically and to generate, within the supervisee, an internal reflective dialogue in which insight and meaning can emerge.

Within supervision, it is therefore important for the supervisor to consider whether an interpretation is focusing on what it is saying or on what it is doing or both. The questions that this raises are:

- Does the interpretation or dialogue provide a degree of uncertainty that allows play, exploration, curiosity and movement within the mind of the supervisee?
- Does the supervisory interpretation emerge from a one-, two- or three-person dynamic?
- Does the interpretation utilize transference and countertransference dynamics in a mutative way and turn what is being presented into reflected objects for the supervisee in relation to the internal world of the patient?
- And, perhaps most importantly, do the words and language of the interpretation take the supervisee to a reflective and insightful place that generates a mutative shift which develops the work with the patient?

From time to time, as supervisors, we probably use a variety of interpretations to facilitate our understanding and reflection of the patient's material. Indeed, there may be other ways in which interpretation can be considered. However, as with any process within therapy and supervision, it is important to consider the dynamics of a process in which it is the response to an interpretation which is of primary importance. It is therefore vital that any consideration of the dynamics and interactions within supervision explores not only what interpretations say but also what they do.

REFERENCES

Bollas C (1991a) The Shadow of the Object. London: Free Association Books.

Bollas C (1991b) Forces of Destiny. London: Free Association Books.

Bollas C (1993) 'The aesthetic moment and the search for transformation'. In Rudnytsky PL (ed.), Transitional Objects and Potential Spaces. New York and Chichester: Columbia University Press.

Caper R (1999) A Mind of One's Own. London and New York: Routledge.

Casement P (1985) On Learning from the Patient. London and New York: Tavistock Publications.

Casement P (1999) Further Learning from the Patient. London: Routledge.

Davies H (2003) Copenhagen. Adapted from the play by Michael Frayn. BBC 2, 30 August 2003.

Fonagy P (2001) Attachment Theory and Psychoanalysis. New York: Other Press.

Fordham M (1986) Interpretation in Jungian Psychotherapy. London: Karnac Books.

Frayn M (2003) Copenhagen. Play adapted for television by Howard Davies. Broadcast on BBC 2, 30 August 2003.

Gee H (1998) 'Developing insight through supervision: relating, then defining'. In Clarkson P (ed.), Supervision, Psychoanalytic and Jungian Perspectives. London: Whurr Publishers.

Heisenberg W (2001) 'Quantum mechanics: Heisenberg uncertainty principle'. In Encyclopaedia Britannica (CD Rom): 1–2.

James W (1901) The Principles of Psychology. Vol 1. London: Macmillan.

James W (1950) The Principles of Psychology. Vol 2. New York: Dover Publications.

Jonte-Pace D (1997) 'Julia Kristeva and the psychoanalytic study of religion: rethinking Freud's cultural texts'. In Jacobs JL, Capps D (eds), Religion, Society and Psychoanalysis. Boulder, CO, and Oxford: Westview Press.

Langs R (1994) Doing Supervision and Being Supervised. London: Karnac Books.

Mander G (1998) 'Dyads and triads: some thoughts on the nature of therapy supervision'. In Clarkson P (ed.), Supervision, Psychoanalytic and Jungian Perspectives. London: Whurr Publishers.

Martin E (2002) 'Listening to the absent patient'. In Driver C, Martin E (eds), Supervising Psychotherapy. London: Sage Publications.

Meltzer D (2003) Supervisions with Donald Meltzer. London and New York: Karnac Books.

Moi T (ed.) (1986) The Kristeva Reader. New York: Columbia University Press.

Monk R (1991) Ludwig Wittgenstein: the Duty of Genius. London: Vintage Press.

Ogden TH (1994) The analytic third: working with intersubjective clinical facts. International Journal Psychoanalysis 75(1): 3–19.

Ogden TH (1999) Reverie and Interpretation. London: Karnac Books.

Piaget J (1958) The Development of Thought: Equilibration of Cognitive Structures. New York: Viking.

Searles HF (1955) 'The informational value of the supervisor's emotional experiences'. In Searles HF (1986) Collected Papers on Schizophrenia and Related Subjects. London: Maresfield Library.

Siegel DJ (1998) The developing mind: toward a neurobiology of interpersonal experience. The Signal: Newsletter of the World Association for Infant Mental Health 6(3–4) July–December: 1–11.

Strachey J (1934) The nature of the therapeutic action of psychoanalysis. International Journal of Psycho-Analysis 15(1): 127–159.

Szecsödy I (1997) '(How) is learning possible in supervision?' In Martindale B et al. (eds), Supervision and its Vicissitudes. London: Karnac Books.

Vygotsky L (2002) Thought and Language. Cambridge, MA, and London: The MIT Press.

Winnicott DW (1980) Playing and Reality. Harmondsworth: Penguin Books.

Wittgenstein L (2001) Philosophical Investigations. Cambridge, MA, and Oxford: Blackwell Publishing.

CHAPTER 3

BION'S 'VERTEX' AS A SUPERVISORY OBJECT

VERNON YORKE

THE PSYCHIC DIMENSION OF SUPERVISION

This chapter is about an aspect of supervision that is not so much concerned with the patient session but is focused more on a particular kind of mind-making in supervisory work. It is predicated on the notion that the more skill and sophistication achieved with this facility in supervision, the greater its availability in work with patients where the creation of mind is paramount. The thinking and practical approaches to work advocated by Bion will form the background for this exploration of how mind is created from what is known, but unknown, within and between the supervisee and supervisor, through the realizing of meaning that can become available for thinking and ultimately understanding.

One of the distractions of supervision is that third-party or one-place-removed reporting tempts us to want to know what's going on, fill gaps, assemble details and reconstruct an accurate and (ostensibly) complete verbatim account. Awkwardly, there remains material not part of the report or the observable session, psychic material that only psychic processes will reveal. To perceive psychic material is not a matter of understanding the words. Words cannot convey the fullness of meaning. Nor is it a matter of the context of other non-verbal features, as we well know from the use of one-way observational mirrors, audio and video recordings and other such attempts to capture human interaction. None of these can reveal these levels of psychic meaning. Audio-visual material is deceptive because we occasionally see meaningful films and television programmes, but they are works of art and not mere recordings of interpersonal interactions. To gain access to meaning there has to be an engagement of minds; only minds can deal in meaning.

PHENOMENOLOGY OF SUPERVISION

In chapter 1 of *Transformations*, Bion (1965) uses the example of a painting of a field of poppies to consider the issue of representation and source material. The field of poppies is the original scene, the fundamental source material, and there is the painter's picture or representation of it. Bion assigns the letter 'O' to refer to source material of any kind because of its truth and its ultimate reality, which cannot be directly known, only partially and indirectly implied and intuitively inferred. That, in a nutshell, is the central difficulty for art and for any process, such as supervision, that deals in representations. Bion refers to these representations of O (the 'picture') as transformations. The picture is not a field of poppies, he observes, but a 'canvas with pigment disposed upon its surface' (Bion 1965: 1). The artist's *work* is the transformation of one to the other, which gives the viewer something of the experience of the field of poppies. The artist's work lies within his mind and his hand, which will condition how he perceives the scene and how he will represent it. Following this analogy, supervision is not a (re)production of the therapeutic session, but one in which the supervisee will always give the supervisor something of the experience of the therapeutic work, provided the supervisor is receptive and able to understand his or her perceptions.

Bion also includes consideration of artistic styles and schools as having a bearing on the transformation. He mentions impressionism and realism as examples. Going into the more abstract schools, a painter like Picasso also includes abstracted and internal dimensions, so that the picture might not even *look* like the source, and may actually contain much more information in the form of a highly sophisticated analysis. Paradoxically, although painting is a visual medium, the subject (O) may in fact never have been 'visible' but only alluded to through the 'picture'. It may be doubtful that we can ever 'know' what the picture is about. What post-realism and abstract approaches to painting achieved was an escape from the tyranny of the subject. In supervision the reconstructed session or the verbatim account can become a similar problem. If such a reconstructed session is regarded as the true subject, this can create a tyranny whereby the unconscious, allusive and invisible communications and meanings remain unrealized.

Post-realism developments suggest that painting has always been allusive and that understanding art is a subjective-intuitive process. Subjective intuitive processes are often mistaken for feeling, but feeling is a rational function of the psyche. The psychic dimension is irrational, and access to it in supervision requires skills with intuitive and irrational methods of working. It is this aspect of supervision – that is, the irrational aspects of the experience with the supervisee – which are the 'royal road' to the exhibition of O as the supervisory object. Its unknowable truth, and ultimate reality, is not accessible merely in the reconstruction.

If pictures are not pictures *of* subjects but pictures *about* subjects, this is not only because of representational processes (transformations) but also because of the way in which they are read in the meeting of minds between viewer and artist. A 'Picasso' is not a picture of something but a piece of Picasso's mind, which requires a piece of ours. In this respect, 'beauty in the eye of the beholder' is not merely an observation about subjectivity but something of the dynamic activity inherent in reading. For Picasso, then, a picture is partly a transformation and potentially a new O; for us it *must* be a new O, and so too the experience in supervision.

In Bion's view, certain features do not change in the process of transformation; he calls them 'invariants', and ordinarily it is these that orient us in understanding what the picture is about. For example, it may be the redness which suggests that these flowers are poppies. When we see a picture or any other work of art, we may not have access to the source material. What we have is the artefact, and we have to decide what it is about. Is the painting *of* a field of poppies, *about* a field of poppies or is the artist (re)presenting something else? This is the predicament of the supervisor, although supervision is not so much like looking at a picture as entering a gallery. In supervision, it may not be clear what the artefact is with which we are to engage. In the gallery too, one is always presented with the problem of which things are the exhibits and which things are parts of the gallery – and whether this matters.

Recently, the Turner Prize was awarded to Martin Creed for a contribution in which the gallery was empty save for a light being switched on and off. Is this art without an artefact? It is, therefore, now possible to engage with a work of art without the necessity to see it or even visit the gallery. In fact, this is possible at any time in the future long after the exhibition has closed. Each viewing is a new experience. This is similar to the state of affairs in supervision: for, while it is strangely oriented upon a re-viewing of past events from elsewhere, it is primarily a live dynamic event in the here and now.

Later in *Transformations*, Bion (1965: 47) draws a distinction between a transformation and a distortion. A distortion is a representation in which the subject O is *misrepresented*. He considers another analogy of the image of some trees seen as a reflection in a lake from the opposite bank. He takes atmospheric effects, or disturbances of the surface of the water, as distortions, which are different from transformations in that a distortion obscures or misrepresents the source data.

O IN SUPERVISION

The O of supervision is unknown. It lies within and between the supervisory participants (supervisor and supervisee(s)) and can therefore have many sources. The patient's O, or source of their material as represented by their transformations, is, in a sense, *no longer theirs*: the therapist's selection of material is independent, a factor of the therapist's mind. It *may* include trans-formations of the patient's transformations, but, since O is unknowable, the patient's transformations as remembered and reported cannot be O in so far as these are conscious elements in the therapist's mind.

The O of supervision will contain links to the patient's transformations in so far as the patient and therapist reach deep into areas of their minds made mutu-ally available for that purpose. In the supervisory situation, the therapist's total contribution (conscious and unconscious) will contain the psychic links to the patient. We can trust this and attend to the supervisory process, which is about the development of a facility for transformations in and of O, without being too tyrannized by the demands of the patient work. Since the O of the supervision is unknown and could lie anywhere in the deeper reaches within and between the supervisory pair and all that they bring, this constitutes a massive array of possibilities. Although this mass of possibilities contains the potential meaning of the supervision, it also poses methodological problems of how to become ori-ented in such an array of material and how to proceed with material of the psychic dimension in order to gain understanding. Bion's legacy contains a methodology suited for proceeding with these matters.

METHODOLOGY

As already stated, the transformational possibilities are infinite. Our conscious intellect is incapable of processing such high volumes of material. It is also unable to process this kind of psychic material because of its *fundamental* nature, in the sense of its rawness. In contrast, the material of consciousness is of an entirely different nature, being comparably more sophisticated. Our conscious minds are formed by, and function on, entirely different principles. We have to turn therefore to the unconscious mind, which does contain processes formed on principles which *are* capable of handling the enormous volume of psychic material, through its ability to compress and generalize psychic material into high-density multidimensional forms and complexes (see Martin, chapter 1; Freud 1955; Matte-Blanco 1975). Here we may turn to Bion's method. This enables the unconscious working of the material of the psychic dimension to be organized and structured in O by using his suggestions to approach the work, first, without memory, desire or understanding (Bion 1967) (further to Freud's rule of abstinence (1958a)) and, second, by entering a state which he calls 'reverie' (Bion 1962) (extending Freud's 1958b 'evenly hovering atten-tion'). Reverie is a state of openness to the dream world where, through its particular principles and psychic processes – for example Freud's 'primary processes' (1955: 460) and 'dream work' (1955: 588) – fundamental source mate-rial (O) is given form, thus ensuring its accessibility.

MEMORY, DESIRE AND UNDERSTANDING

To be without memory, desire and understanding is about having an open mind, and a cleared mind. There are at least two good reasons for adopting this position. First of all, as Bion observed, the time of the session exists as the only opportunity one has to observe the session to see what is there. To go into supervision with memories, desires, things already known or thought to be, hopes, fears, expectations or any other kinds of agenda all present obstacles to the clear observation of the phenomena one is witnessing and is part of. Such agendas will create serious disturbances on 'the lake' (distortions) and obscure and deflect the exploration, preventing the realization of the supervisory object.

Second, an attachment to memories, desires and understandings locks one into a conscious attitude, where all the possibilities are already replete with old meaning with no venue for any new material to occupy. Not only can nothing new be observed but also no new meanings can be discovered, no new ideas, mind, content or structure. The state of reverie is a state of unfulfilled receptivity: an emotional preparedness and venue for psychic meaning in the form of rising intuition: new food for new thought and new understanding.

However, if memories and desires are evoked in supervision, they are part of the supervision and should be regarded as valid material. Indeed, it is such evocations rising in the reverie that *will* lead to a key to understanding the potential meanings within the supervisory situation. The 'key' is a particular idea that emerges out of the reverie state, which binds the material together in a new way that integrates it into a particular sense. Bion borrowed the term 'selected fact' for this binding and integrating function from the philosopher Henri Poincaré (1952). Initially, it comes as an intuition: knowledge with rhyme but no reasons. The reasons and meanings will be consequent developments.

REVERIE AND THE SELECTED FACT

Reverie is a deceptively simple term that describes the deliberate and necessary suspension of conscious processes in favour of unconscious processes. It is achieved through the activity of clearing the mind by the suspension of memories, desires and understandings as outlined above, which opens the mind to a preparedness for states of reverie. So not only is the suspension of memory and desire etc. an attitude, it is also a process with an outcome: a readiness for states of reverie. The phenomenology of reverie can be anything and everything which comes to mind in the supervisory situation: associations and ideas, however vague or fleeting. It may develop into a particular sort of daydream. However, it is important to differentiate between reverie and similar phenomena, for example daydreams or memory. The difference is a technical one where reverie is defined by the possibility of a selected fact. Memories and daydreams may play a role in reverie, but alone are not sufficient.

Typical of the experience of reverie is that while the supervisee is making their presentation the supervisor may become engrossed in a preoccupying interlude which has captured his or her mind. This may be either fleetingly or completely, and may or may not seem related to the current considerations in the supervision. It may be intensely personal. It may be embarrassing, shameful or psychopathological, or seem trivial in content. The initial impulse may be to dismiss it as neurotic countertransference. However, having been immersed, to a greater or lesser extent, in this preoccupation, at a particular point there is a return to the 'surface', that is the supervision in progress, and perhaps accompanied by some inkling of the relevance and meaningfulness in the daydreaming. This is realized more fully when the interlude, and all of its associated thoughts and feelings, is reviewed and considered alongside what's gone before and how it fits with the current material. Gradually, some ideas begin to gain prominence. They may still seem to have little relevance to the supervisory material until something happens that draws them together into a striking idea which then becomes a key to the understanding of the material.

This initially intuitive realization is the experience of the selected fact. It is the point at which the unconscious work crosses over into consciousness and is then available for conscious thought and thinking processes. This means that the material has been suitably transformed in both a form and content that consciousness is equipped to process. The initial intuitions are subject to the rational processes of feeling that ascribe value, and it is this that enables ideas to gather prominence and the selected fact to emerge. After the realization of the selected fact, further work is required, in relation to all the material in the supervision and the supervisor's own mind, as an understanding of ideas emerges and forms in relation to the supervision. Relevant memories and desires of past material may now seem comprehensible in the light of this new material and can become part of the current analysis.

The ideas are also accompanied by the relevant and necessary theoretical frameworks required to think about them. This is an equally important function as there now exists a greater body of common theory and clinical practice, as the demarcation between the various schools of thought lessens in the modern climate of tolerance and institutional intercourse. There is also the added volume as new theory and method are discovered, and old ones extended. This potential for eclecticism is another massive array of material and is naturally contained and structured by O, in the same way as the psychic dimension of the material.

This state of reverie may sound as if one is not paying attention to the supervisee. But, as the process of reverie is run on the principles and rules of unconscious processes, as indicated above, which includes the processing of large volumes and a capability with multidimensional forms, these facilities, unsurprisingly, permit multi-tasking. This means that while one has been seemingly engrossed in reverie one has also been unconsciously listening to and even participating in the discussion in the room. Consequently, nothing is missed. It may take some time and experience in the method before full trust in this process becomes established.

THE VERTEX

This selected particular configuration of ideas and theories becomes a mental position from which one operates as a base. This is similar to how Bion (1965) describes the vertex, although he certainly does not define it in this way. Bion's use of the term vertex almost has, at times, a sense of being a generalized category, for example the religious, psychoanalytic, adult and orthodox are all vertices, yet he also talks about their 'representing views with which I am identified' (Bion 1965: 145). Clearly, they are not an objective point, as the term in its geometric sense means. It cannot be outside or not part of the mind. It is composed of ideas and other mental elements, and forms a basis for consideration and approach.

The term is commonly translated as 'point of view', in the sense of something seen from a particular vantage point, or even better from several different vantage points (Meltzer 1986). While this is true enough, what is being proposed here is that it implies a structure of related ideas that contains meaning and generates the formation of opinion and belief – in other words, mind itself. The vertex is a transformation of O and creates a mental and intellectual (theoretical) position from which to regard the supervisory task. The realization of this O is what is required to take a position in the supervision. It is the supervisory object.

It is impossible to separate these aspects of this creative process and the way in which meaning is released to become mind. The vertex as mind is a detailed and structured exhibition in consciousness of what was the compressed, dense, multidimensional material transformed during the unconscious process of reverie. Unconscious process means we cannot know about it but that we can trust it as true, and real. The selected fact has been described above as the experiential point at which the process crosses the threshold into consciousness. It indicates that it has achieved the necessary conditions (structure and form) for work on it to be continued in consciousness now through a further process of association, amplification and thinking. The vertex is the result of this process: we come to know what we think. We have an opinion, a piece of mind. A vertex is capable of becoming a new O, of becoming immersed in new reveries. One can see here a complex commerce of vertices, immersing and arising out of transformations of

O (reverie) creating new vertices in a progress through more sophisticated forms (growth), as described graphically on Bion's grid (1989).

On the grid, Bion uses different terminology for the phenomena. The source materials are called beta elements, and these may become alpha elements, similar to transformations, via an assumed psychic process he calls alpha function. Alpha elements are suitable for developing into material that can eventually become conscious. The grid was intended as a conceptual tool rather than a model, hence he was at great pains not to ascribe any clinical details to alpha function, or the elements. In the grid, he avoided any analogies, for example to painting as a 'function' in art or poppies as 'elements' in a picture. He envisaged that the grid could be applied to any clinical data, in relation to any hypothetical psychological functions, that any future researcher may imagine.

Application

Having outlined the method in terms of Bion's theoretical and methodological framework, some examples demonstrating its use will now be presented. I would like to consider three particular circumstances to which these psychic tools may be applied in supervision. First, how to foster the method in supervisees and particularly trainees. Second, its use in creating a deeper understanding of the psychic situation in the supervision of patient work and, third, its application to the supervisory relationship.

1: Fostering

It is better to introduce new methods of working in a practical way rather than from a theoretical point of view. Explaining in theory what one might do sets up unhelpful expectations and external criteria. However, by focusing on any fragment of countertransference fantasy, the supervisor utilizes and reflects on something already happening that has an established internal dimension. Everything necessary for understanding already exists in the supervisee's unconscious. The supervisory task is making it available, opening a channel of communication with unconscious processes and creating a venue to think about it.

> This task of opening a channel of communication was clearly illustrated by one supervisee who had a strong sense that his patient's difficulty was represented in the single image of a fairy-tale character but did not know how to move forward from there. The use of this kind of mythical material for amplification is seemingly advocated in Freud's use of the myths of Oedipus and Narcissus, for example. The difficulty with this approach

is that the facts of the myth are dominant and confine one to the parameters of the myth. Bion's brilliant addition to the method of the selected
fact enables one to escape from the myth having found a principle that
orients and orders the material. The selected fact may arise out of the
myth but not actually be part of it. In this case, it was unlocked in supervision by his fleeting mention of a pose struck by a partner which was
nothing to do with the story. Helping him to arrest and explore this
'fleeting image' enabled him to let it organize the *relevant* details in the
fairy tale for him and lead him to the unlikely but revolutionary vertex
that this particular Sleeping Beauty wasn't ready to wake up yet, his initial idea being to wake her and possibly replicate aspects of the rude
awakening by sexual abuse in her childhood. This new vertex did not
violate her developmental position in the transference, and enabled him
to steer a course that did support her development.

The slightest thing – a remark, an image, an attitude, a word – is a possible
golden opportunity. Often these are throw-aways or intrusions to be dismissed
to clear the ground to get back to the 'real' material. I encourage supervisees
to linger on these proto-reveries and pay ever more attention to them. Often
personal associations and details need to be included, and the supervisor has to
be really sure in handling this in a supervisory rather than an analytic way, that
is, looking for the collating principle in the reverie, the meaning for the supervision, rather than exploring the coexisting personal meaning, which would be
a gross intrusion.

> A second example occurred when a supervisee commented that he went
> into a session filled with excitement about a date he had later that
> evening and was relieved when the patient was able to get his attention
> off this and onto him. I suggested the opposite, that he revisit his feelings
> about his date in so far as they were part of the session. It was not long
> before he realized that he had hoped that the patient would cancel, as he
> had done the night before, so that he could meet his date a little earlier.
> This made other material about a missed session, and an imminent holi-
> day break, more ample and able to be understood more fully.

Picking up on these nascent reveries and attempting to find a selected fact
is not only a way one can get behind a supervisee's reverie and support it but
also to encourage some confidence in their psychopathology. This is essential
for work in the area of O, because of its intensely subjective nature. It is particularly important with trainees who have usually had it drummed into them
that their own preoccupations are part of the neurotic countertransference and

must be excluded. It may well be part of the neurotic countertransference, but that doesn't rule it out. It needs simultaneous understanding from two points of view: its place in the work and its place in the therapist's mind, particularly if it is unconscious. If it is conscious, it is not neurotic countertransference. A skilled handling of this delicate balance is one of the professional responsibilities of the supervisor.

2: Reaching deeper psychic material

The beauty of Bion's method is that it advances directly to the deeper levels of the psyche, where it engages with the more fundamental meanings from which the more apparently conscious phenomena draw their motives and driving forces. The supervisor can use the method to discover what meanings are available and energized in the vicinity of the supervision in order to orient him- or herself in relation to helping the supervisee to explore this field and become familiar with the practice of discovering meanings in this way, and how this might facilitate their therapeutic work.

This use of the method by the supervisor is illustrated in the following example. A supervisee talked, in supervision, about a patient with whom she had worked with great care and patience for many years. He was a man who had made remarkable progress with her from the most unlikely prognosis. Among the themes she brought about the patient were:

1. He had to cancel a session by arrangement at the end of the week due to a professional commitment, which made an unusually long gap between his last session and the current one.
2. A new friend had inexplicably and completely blanked him when he'd run into him in an unexpected situation.
3. A relationship of over two years, which he had formed with a woman and felt was going well, and about which he had harboured much hope for the future, had recently been ended by her rather abruptly and very painfully.
4. He found himself suddenly a 'sad old bachelor' and, as the prospect horrifies him, he feels he must do something about it. He sometimes solicits street prostitutes on his way to and from his sessions, and usually when he was on his way to visit his ladyfriend. Since the relationship has ended, this activity has reached what he feels are alarming levels and defines him as the sad old man.
5. He has taken on a major project at work and feels he is out of his depth and that he needs guidance, which is not forthcoming. (In fact, he is extremely capable and well thought of but always underestimates his ability and is amazed when his work is commended.)

The supervisee described, during the supervision, how the patient had arrived extremely angry having walked round the block several times and was visibly on the verge of tears, which was utterly unheard of for him as he would consider that a weakness. She went on to describe how, when the patient was talking about a gravely ill relative and the friend who blanked him, she went off into what she described as a very vivid fantasy. In her fantasy thoughts, she knew there were two eggs in her kitchen and that she 'really fancied an egg mayonnaise sandwich'. She considered tuna mayonnaise as an alternative but decided, 'No, the eggs.' She fantasized preparing it, and the experience was so vivid that she could smell it and taste it, and she added that it was like an hallucination. She then found herself wondering why she was thinking about such things and surfaced to find him saying that he didn't know what he was talking about and had forgotten the point he was trying to make.

Her associations were that she thought that it was in some way about feeding him a kind of children's food, warm and comforting which had a particular 'slurpy' texture (in the food design trade this is known as 'mouth feel'). She felt that she probably rejected tuna mayonnaise on the grounds that it seemed a more sophisticated food. As soon as she finished the session, the idea of an egg mayonnaise sandwich did not appeal to her in the least. It was then that she felt it was particularly the property of the session.

Her account of what the patient was talking about at the points when she 'went off' and came back seemed to me to be seamless and complete rather than having something missing. Although she was concerned that she was not listening to him, and felt sure she'd missed something important, I suspect that this is an example of the multi-tasking suggested above. However, what did seem to 'bring her back' was his disorientation and confusion, as he may have experienced her reverie as an abandonment and may have prevented her from completing the process of releasing the meaning.

In this interlude no selected fact arose; there was just the reverie. With no binding idea, the reverie was in consciousness in much the same way as a dream: vivid, symbolic and pregnant. It lacked focus, rendering it unavailable for thought but was full of possibilities. However, the selected fact doesn't just herald the arrival of the material in consciousness but also, and significantly, orients by providing a heading. It says what the material is about. An important task, at this stage, was to try to facilitate her discovery of her selected fact.

An initial exploration of her associations wandered around in the content: two eggs, mashing and merging, mayonnaise as a binding function, itself made from eggs etc., but while this was all fascinating none of it set us alight. What we lacked was a selected fact that would focus and draw some of this material together. During this exploration, I found myself in my own vivid reverie to do with a memory from when I was about nineteen and working in a provincial theatre where the night security staff had a guard dog. During the interval, a large container of coffee was sent backstage for the scene-shifters. A few of us usually drank some and the rest, possibly half a gallon or so, was put down for the dog. The dog would begin to lap it up and then after a while would start to growl, bark and whimper while it continued to drink as if enraged by the pan of coffee. This strange behaviour of the dog was a matter of much amusement to the security men. Plainly, the dog was drinking that amount every day and had acquired a serious addiction to caffeine. I surfaced back into the supervision with the selected fact of addiction as the centrally binding idea and began to review the interlude and all else besides. I began to think about the material in the following way.

The patient, probably provoked by the longer gap between the sessions, had almost become aware of his dependence, which he may experience as 'reeling him in' as he walks round the block. He was furious to find himself in this position. He was possibly bewildered as to how it got to this state of affairs in view of the fact that he had taken the precaution to keep his appetite away from his therapist by his pre- and post-session attempts to arrive already satisfied or to be careful to take his hunger out with him for satisfaction elsewhere. In the way that the dog was enraged about the volume of the coffee which it did not want but had to have to be able to get the caffeine it craved, this man finds himself in a dangerous situation with his therapist which he does not want but has to have in order to have her know him and understand him. He needs this more than anything. He has never had this before and fears that he has or will become addicted to it. The danger is that he is out of his depth, he will not be enough for her, she may now blank him, end the relationship, become terminally ill and abandon him.

I regard all this as background orientation against which to proceed with supervision rather than offering it as a possible version because I am not wanting merely to understand the therapeutic material but to try and discover a way of engaging with the supervisee's reverie. Using only my selected fact, I said that I wondered if it had something to do with addiction. She then took off with the comment that he doesn't like all his 'eggs in one basket', how he has always had other alternative therapies and people he consulted in the wings, but this had gradually fallen off and she was beginning to look like the only person in the picture and certainly the only one who had endured. She remembered that he had reduced his sessions because he was worried about dependence. In the session, she had wondered whether he wanted to increase the number of sessions again but thought that this would have to come from him and wondered whether he would ask for this. She'd also thought about the summer holiday and that he would expect her to tell him about it around now. She recalled that last year she'd had to take a much longer break for personal and family reasons and that perhaps he was anticipating a similar announcement. It wasn't long before we were having a deep and wide-ranging discussion about all this and more, which had life and conviction.

While I used my reverie implicitly to understand the material and create a focus, I only used it explicitly to re-engage her with her reverie and lead to *her* selected fact ('eggs in one basket'). I also kept her reverie at the heart of the supervision with its links to the therapeutic material, from which she derived different conclusions more accurate than mine. This is not only important but desirable as it is the supervisee who has to carry authenticity and conviction into the work, and is much better than second-hand ideas from her supervisor, however impressive they may look.

By responding in kind, and engaging with her experience in this way, a new level of working in supervision opened up for us. If the therapeutic work is better understood, and the patient is the beneficiary of it, this is a happy bonus. We have a lot more work to do in honing this particular method from which this and other patients may hopefully benefit. This way of working certainly has a greater range and depth than confining ourselves to trying to understand a particular countertransference fantasy on a Thursday afternoon.

3: The supervisory relationship

Supervision is a close and often long-term professional relationship. However, while it is about analytic principles, it is not explicitly conducted on those principles, in the same way as psychotherapy. Nevertheless, difficulties can and do arise in the relationship, which may affect the therapeutic work, and difficulties in the work certainly affect the supervisory relationship, a phenomenon well known as the parallel process. The supervisor needs to be aware of many factors within the supervisee's progress in order to make the professional judgements that one has to make as a supervisor at various points. The method based on Bion's ideas proposed here is a useful supervisory tool for assessing many of the deeper aspects of the supervisory relationship, as the following example illustrates.

This supervisee was terminating with his patient, owing to events in the therapist's life, and they had been working through quite a long period of notice. The patient had been working quite well through this difficult period, to some good effect. A month before the end, during our supervision, I found myself with a detailed memory of having been abandoned in the rain by a woman and my car having been towed away during a visit to the cinema to see the film *The Omen*. My anger and disappointment were as alive in this interlude as if it were yesterday. Equally alive, I remembered knowing that our relationship was coming apart, and, although I wanted her, I also knew that I was not the kind of man that she wanted. I had tried to remain philosophical about it and accept that I had been abandoned and be graceful about it rather than pursue a futile suit.

I rejoined the supervision, from my thoughts, to a point where the supervisee was describing how the patient had started to say mysterious things and had been asking very particular but mysterious questions, about the therapist's future. The supervisee then revealed that events had taken a very different and unexpected turn and in fact the termination was no longer necessary. However, he felt that it was too late to turn back now and that they must press on to the end.

I attempted an examination of the vertex from my material, but the strong set of feelings that I was having were that the therapy had not run its proper course and was being truncated and that it would remain a sadly unfinished project which would have finished successfully had it run its natural course. I said to the supervisee that there seemed to be a lot of things in this that had not been thought about, adding a comment that a resumption must not be ruled out, however unlikely or undesirable such a reversal might be.

The next meeting was filled with ambivalence about the end, some intense anger from the patient and some attempts to resuscitate the erotic aspects of the transference relationship in the face of all this. Although I was impressed with the emotional tenacity of the patient, I remained unsure. I again reiterated my comment that there were issues which remained unthought about.

The next supervisory meeting contained spectacular material of the mourning of the loss and how, for the patient, it was worse than a death because the therapist was still here. Other emotional material was impressive in its maturity and courage and the refusal to take an easy distraction. In particular, there was also an evaluation of the loss of past significant relationships. I could see that this patient had not only managed to engage fully with the end but was completing the project which I had described as unnaturally truncated. Equally significantly, the therapist interacted with the patient's material with sensitive resonance, while containing some narcissistic impulses and sexual longings that he saw as potentially crippling this patient were he not to 'let her go'. The candour without 'spillage' was admirable.

Being clearly so wrong, I had to re-examine my flawed 'thinking'(though it is more properly a pocket of mindlessness) and was then able to also see that the unthought issue was the ending of our supervision. Indeed, there was no real selected fact, only some strong feelings. My reverie had become perverted into a memory, which distorted and obscured the meaning of the supervision. Also, my attention was deflected from the supervisory object onto the patient work, which at that point became the subject of a rather tyrannical desire. I thought I 'knew' that the therapeutic work was not running its natural course, and this obscured the fact that the theme of completion belonged in the supervision. Another desire, a retrospective one, was that my relationship with the woman from the past would have been successful had it run its natural course. In fact, it *had* run its natural course! As had the therapy, and particularly the supervision. All this memory, desire and understanding, was summoned under the pressures of abandonment and other dynamics in the supervisory relationship. It was this we wished to remain gracefully 'philosophical' about, that is blissfully unconscious about, as well as ignorant of, our angers and disappointments regarding the end of the supervision.

This had been a long and very satisfying supervisory relationship both in the progress of the supervisee and the patient as well as myself. It was a lot to lose, and we had not really addressed this matter. Acknowledging our ending provoked a very intense emotional moment between us. Apart from its emotional face value, this also served as a symbol for something that feels too deep to negotiate and was almost evaded. Perhaps that is always true in greater or lesser measure in every ending, but never any lesser in meaning.

There were difficulties for the supervisee highlighted by these themes, which he had to examine in himself. There is no need for an excursion into that, since the focus here is more the supervisor's inner process, but it was by no means a one-sided matter.

An important aspect of this flaw in my supervision was that the therapist disagreed with me and did not panic or change direction, even under some pressure from me. I am not sure I could have held as firm as he did had I been in his position. I had asked him to think about it, and he did; he decided to proceed. His internal strength was a factor in enabling the patient to feel supported into the mourning. He clearly had his own mind, a reliable object he could trust. This made it abundantly clear that the supervision was in a good position to end, not because his patient was leaving but because he had arrived at a natural point. I cannot claim that this was my intention. Here the realization of the supervisory object came about in an extraordinary way, but nevertheless a very real one. However, the need for discipline in regard to the accurate identification of the selected fact cannot be overemphasized. The temptation to self-indulgence in the reverie is one of the risks inherent in the method.

CONCLUSION

Supervision is concerned with a particular kind of mind-making from which a sound professional identity is created. Some supervisory tools have been suggested that may prove to be interesting and useful. They are based on some of Bion's ideas about discipline, freedom and courage: discipline in observation and in the supervisor's state of mind, freedom in the search for a subject and plumbing one's own depths and courage to engage and not evade the meaning that might be found there. Courage too for deep psychic engagement with the supervisee, while forgoing the comfort of rank and status. Without this engagement, the meaning of the supervision may be lost, as meaning can only be realized through mind. Supervision is a meeting of minds, enabled by skills with irrational psychic processes

Bion's concept of the vertex has been used as a pivotal point in the growth of ideas as it stands at the end point of a transformational process where something has been known that simultaneously implies something which remains unknown. The concept has also been pressed into the role of container for the artificial but helpful notion of a supervisory object. It enables us to draw a meaningful line, which enables us to draw breath as we make our way in a universe of possibilities.

REFERENCES

Bion WR (1962) A Theory of Thinking. International Journal of Psycho-Analysis 43(4): 306–310.
Bion WR (1965) Transformations. London: Heinemann.
Bion WR (1967) Notes on Memory and Desire. Psycho Analytic Forum 2(3): 272–273.
Bion WR (1989) Two Papers: the Grid and Caesura. London: Karnac Books.
Freud S (1955) The Interpretation of Dreams. SE 5. London: Hogarth Press.
Freud S (1958a) Case History of Schreber, Papers on Technique and Other Works. SE 12: 165. London: Hogarth Press.
Freud S (1958b) Recommendations to Physicians Practicing Psychoanalysis. SE 12. London: Hogarth Press.
Matte-Blanco I (1975) The Unconscious as Infinite Sets. London: Duckworth.
Meltzer DM (1986) Studies in Extended Metapsychology. Perthshire: Clunie Press.
Poincaré H (1952) Science and Method. New York: Dover Publications.

Chapter 4

Free association and supervision

Stephen Crawford

Introduction

Saul Bellow's novel *Ravelstein* revolves around the friendship between two American intellectuals, at a time when their wide-ranging conversations are becoming overshadowed by the illness and approaching death of the character who gives the novel its name. The novel's narrator reports how Ravelstein asked him what he imagined death would be like, and how he answered that 'the pictures would stop' (Bellow 2001: 222). This answer expresses, in very simple language, something important about the way people experience the workings of their own minds, namely that there is activity, an ebb and flow of thoughts, memories, perceptions and sensations. For some people, this activity may be highly visual, and aptly described as 'pictures', while for others it may be less so. It almost certainly will not be constant, and at times may appear to stop. Nonetheless, it is hard to imagine there being no thoughts, or pictures, while a person is alive and in good health.

This certainly seems to be the view of Bellow's narrator, for whom life means pictures while death means the end of thought, of consciousness and of experience. He suggests that we are so attached to our own consciousness that we find it hard to really believe that it ever dies: 'I wonder if anyone believes that the grave is all there is. No one can give up on the pictures' (Bellow 2001: 222). From a psychoanalytic perspective, this is the subject's narcissism speaking, expressing disbelief that the world could carry on without them.

What I am seeking to highlight here is the centrality in our lives of the activity of mind, as a way of introducing the notion of free association and of indicating why it is so important in psychoanalysis. This is not to say that mental life consists only of free association. It is possible to classify thought into different kinds, each with differing emphases or purposes. In their study of supervision, Jacobs et al. (1995) examine four forms of thinking which they consider to be necessary to the practice of therapy and also of supervision. These are associative, inductive, creative and self-reflective modes of thought. Inductive thought is to do with reasoning and the framing of hypotheses, while creative and self-reflective thought are reasonably self-explanatory. Associative thought, 'the joining of one thought with another without an immediate conscious goal' (Jacobs et al. 1995: 77), is the subject of this chapter, and, although only one of their four categories, Jacobs et al. do underline the importance of associative thinking in mental life by describing it as 'the fabric of all thought' (Jacobs et al. 1995: 85).

I will now consider Freud's introduction of the concept of free association, then go on to look at how some other writers in the psychoanalytic tradition have developed the concept, before exploring the relevance of free association to supervision.

FREUD AND FREE ASSOCIATION

When Freud introduced free association into psychoanalysis, I think he did so believing that mental activity is a given, both when we are awake and also, of course, when we are asleep and dream. Freud's interest was in what might lie beneath the thoughts present to consciousness and in the nature of the forces at work in the mind that are able to make some thoughts unconscious, and keep them so.

According to Laplanche and Pontalis (1973), Freud developed the method of free association between 1892 and 1898, drawing among other things on his experiences as reported in the *Studies on Hysteria* (Freud and Breuer 1895) and on his own self-analysis, particularly the analysis of his own dreams (Laplanche and Pontalis 1973: 169–170). The basic idea of the method is quite simple, as Freud makes clear in his paper *On Beginning the Treatment* (1913), where he also gives a memorable image of how the patient should think of themselves:

> *You will notice that as you relate things various thoughts will occur to you which you would like to put aside on the ground of certain criticisms and objections. You will be tempted to say to yourself that this or that is irrelevant here, or is quite unimportant, or nonsensical, so that there is no need to say it. You must never give in to these criticisms, but must say it in spite of them – indeed, you must say it precisely because you feel an aversion to doing so. Later on you will find out and learn to understand the reason for this injunction, which is really the only one you have to follow. So say whatever goes through your mind. Act as though, for instance, you were a traveller sitting next to the window of a railway carriage and describing to someone inside the carriage the changing views which you see outside. Finally, never forget that you have promised to be absolutely honest, and never leave anything out because, for some reason or other, it is unpleasant to tell it.*   (Freud 1913: 134–135)

For Freud, the method of free association followed from his theory of the repressed unconscious and the idea that thoughts under repression continue to try and gain access to consciousness but can only do so in disguised forms. It is these disguised substitutes that will emerge in the patient's free associations, provided that the patient follows the 'fundamental rule' of psychoanalysis, by saying everything that comes into his mind. At the same time, however, Freud also says that 'free association is not really free' (Freud 1925: 224), in that the 'patient remains under the influence of the analytic situation even though he is not directing his mental activities on to a particular subject' (Freud 1925: 224), so that the associations that emerge will have a connection back to the repressed thoughts that underlie the difficulties that have brought the patient to analysis.

Just as the patient must agree to the method of free association, Freud recommends a complementary approach for the therapist:

> *Experience soon showed that the attitude that the analytic physician could most advantageously adopt was to surrender himself to his own unconscious mental activity, in a state of evenly suspended attention, to avoid so far as possible reflection and the construction of conscious expectations, not to try and fix anything that he heard particularly in his memory, and by these means to catch the drift of the patient's unconscious with his own unconscious.*   (Freud 1923: 136)

Following from this, Freud warns against the dangers of the analyst making a conscious selection from the patient's material, on the grounds that to do so would be to follow his own expectations, or inclinations, rather than be open to the patient's unconscious meaning. He also warns against any idea that the patient's meaning might be open to an immediate understanding, saying that 'the things one hears are for the most part things whose meaning is only recognised later on' (Freud 1912: 112). Put rather bluntly, the analyst 'should simply listen, and not bother about whether he is keeping anything in mind' (Freud 1912: 112). For Freud, 'the work of analysis involves an art of interpretation' (Freud 1925: 224), and the ideas that form the basis of interpretation arise out of the practice of 'evenly suspended attention'.

One further significant element in Freud's writing about free association is his use of two different expressions in the original German text. In the phrase *'freie Assoziation'*, *Assoziation* 'refers to elements composing a chain – either the chain of logical argument or a chain of those associations which, though described as free, are nonetheless determined' (Laplanche and Pontalis 1973: 178). In this case, the determination of the associations arises from the unconscious, not from conscious selection. In addition, Freud also uses the word *'Einfall'*, 'literally what falls into the mind' (Laplanche and Pontalis 1973: 178), to designate 'all the ideas that come to the subject in the course of the analytic session, even where the associative links underlying them are not apparent, and even where they appear subjectively as unconnected with the context' (Laplanche and Pontalis 1973: 178). In other words, although Freud can seem insistent on the idea of determination, or, that the 'arbitrary has no existence in mental life' (Freud 1909: 261), his use of *Einfall* allows him to preserve the subjective experience of having an idea that seems to come out of the blue.

FREE ASSOCIATION IN PSYCHOANALYSIS SINCE FREUD

Free association has retained a central place in psychoanalytic practice since it was first introduced by Freud. Indeed, one analyst recently suggested that what 'unites our pluralistic, divided discipline is a commitment to the free association method and its meaning' (Williams 2002: 471). It has not, however, been without controversy, and there has been an ongoing discussion about what exactly it is. Freud's account of free association makes it clear that there will be resistances in the way of free associating, and that transference may become a particular form of resistance (Freud 1925: 225). But, over time, there has developed a tendency among analysts to 'regard free association as a distant and unrealisable ideal' (Bollas 2002: 9), as if no one in analysis could free associate in any meaningful way, and, if they could, they would no longer need to be in analysis. For Freud, it seems that free association gives the analyst enough material to go on to begin an approach to what was unconscious through interpretation. However, following his formulation of the structural model of ego, id and superego (Freud 1923), and the development of this model by his daughter Anna, by ego psychologists in the United States and by others working in the psychoanalytic tradition, more attention has been given to how the ego's mechanisms of defence and the superego both contribute to restricting free association (Freud 1936; Mitchell and Black 1995: 27).

It seems that there is still a tension between analysts like Bollas, who suggests redefining free association as *'free talking*, as nothing more than talking about what is on the mind, moving from one topic to another in a free-moving sequence that does not follow an agenda' (Bollas 2002: 9), and those like Williams, for example, who, emphasizing the restrictions on free association, writes that much 'present day psychoanalytic work is dedicated to understanding forms of negative therapeutic reaction to free association, particularly through the examination of mutations of the superego' (Williams 2002: 473). The tension almost seems to be between trying to follow and work with what free association there is, on the one hand, versus concentrating on understanding and interpreting the limitations and restrictions in the way of free association on the other. Perhaps the question is whether what is *not* said is more significant than what *is* said, or not, although I suspect that most therapists will be working in both ways. I now want to highlight some particular contributions to thinking about free association since Freud.

Winnicott makes some remarks about free association in his paper *Playing: Creative Activity and the Search for the Self* (Winnicott 1985b). By this time in his work, he had developed his theory of the true self and the associated idea of the spontaneous gesture, a creative act arising from the self's initiative rather than as a reaction to impingement, or outside influence. In its turn, the emergence of the true self depended on the good-enough adaptation of the mother or principal carer of the baby during the phase of absolute dependence at the beginning of post-natal life. Winnicott seems to see an analogy between the spontaneous gesture and some forms of free association. He writes:

> In the relaxation that belongs to trust and to acceptance of the professional reliability of the therapeutic setting . . . there is room for the idea of unrelated thought sequences which the analyst will do well to accept as such, not assuming the existence of a significant thread . . . According to this theory, free association that reveals a coherent theme is already affected by anxiety, and the cohesion of ideas is a defence organisation.   (Winnicott 1985b: 65)

In this statement, Winnicott clearly links one kind of free association with anxiety and defence, saying that it is these that make the associations coherent. In contrast, he does also have an idea of 'unrelated thought sequences', reminiscent of Freud's *Einfall*, which may or may not reveal a significant thread of connection. Although he does not spell it out, I think he is making room for the patient's spontaneous gesture manifesting as an 'unrelated thought sequence', in the analytic setting. Unlike Freud, I think Winnicott wants to leave open the possibility of thoughts that might be relatively free from determination although arising out of the character and experience of a particular personality. Like Freud, there seems to be an acceptance that a patient's meaning may not be immediately clear and may only emerge in time.

Winnicott, more than anyone else in the psychoanalytic tradition, has written about the importance of play, not least for what it allows of the true self's expression. While I do not think Freud would have envisaged free association in itself as play, I think that Winnicott's ideas about psychotherapy being '*to do with two people playing together*' (Winnicott 1985a: 44) are relevant to the practice of free association: therapist and patient engaged in a to-and-fro process in which each may contribute to the exploration and development of a theme.

Kris writes extensively about free association and conceives of it as:

> . . . a joint venture in which the patient attempts to express whatever comes to mind, that is, the free associations, and the analyst, guided by his own associations and formulations, contributes only with the goal of enhancing the expression of the patient's free associations, expanding the patient's freedom of association.   (Kris 1996: 3)

For Kris, the method of free association is 'the product of two minds at work' (Kris 1996: ix), and no doubt Winnicott might want to add 'and at play'. I think that this idea is a logical extension of Freud's description of the free-associating patient in relation to the analyst in the state of evenly suspended attention. Kris, like Bollas, also seems of the view that free association is not an unapproachable ideal but rather 'the ordinary stuff of everyday life' (Kris 1996: 8) and that the capacity to associate can be developed and that such development has therapeutic value in its own right, as well as by virtue of what it reveals.

A group of papers published in the *British Journal of Psychotherapy* that were given at a conference on 'Free Association and the Unconscious' focus on the difficulties and limitations in free association (Bronstein 2002; Garland 2002; Mawson 2002; Williams 2002) but also highlight how association as a concept can be extended to include communications from the patient that are non-verbal, and which the therapist may be able to process and put into words. Williams, for example, writes about the emotional and bodily discomfort a therapist may feel in the presence of a patient using primitive defences involving projection. He writes:

> ... I would argue that these patients are associating to their internal world, but not in any sense that could be said to be free, differentiated or collaborative. They experience rudimentary, psycho-physiological rejoinders to internal and external events, and these reactions bypass thought or reflection. This is why the analyst must be attentive to the rudimentary character and its latent, yet-to-be-symbolised meaning.
>
> (Williams 2002: 475)

These authors are also interested in questions of how much freedom both patient and analyst can be allowed, to think their own thoughts and communicate with each other about what each may have said or be imagined to be thinking. As Bronstein notes, there will be times of greater 'fluidity' in a patient's associations but also times when the therapist experiences the patient as trying to control both what is said and what can be thought (Bronstein 2002: 479).

For Garland, there is an important Oedipal dimension to free association in the sense of how much freedom can the significant others in a person's life be given to be in relationship with each other as well as with the subject. In the Oedipal situation, the child is seen as desiring the love and presence of one parent, while wanting to keep the other at a distance and treating them as a rival. As a result, it is seen as an achievement if and when the child can tolerate the relationship that exists between the parents and which to some extent excludes the child. Garland suggests 'that "free association" in a modern analysis can be taken usefully to include the way a patient links up with – associates with – his or her objects, internally and externally' (Garland 2002: 491) and that development in therapy may involve a 'growing capacity to allow . . . *objects to associate freely with each other*' (Garland 2002: 508). These ideas have a particular significance to supervision, which I shall return to below.

Bollas' short book *Free Association* emphasizes the possibilities and potentials of free associating rather than the obstacles to, and restrictions on, it. His approach is both sophisticated and down to earth. As I have said, he suggests using the term 'free talking' in order to get away from an idealized view of free association that has developed since Freud (Bollas 2002: 9). He links free association with creativity and with what he calls 'the human drive to represent' (Bollas 2002: 60), in a way that Winnicott would, I think, have agreed with, and suggests that free associating 'enhances the patient's unconscious reach' (Bollas 2002: 40) and enables 'the development of unconscious capabilities' (Bollas 2002: 66).

For Bollas, free association is an expansive process that can contribute to the development of the mind. It may occur according to the 'logic of sequence', in other words, Freud's idea of associative chains spreading in multiple directions, or the 'logic of projection', namely the understanding developed by Klein and object-relations theorists of the importance of projective processes in mental life and in communication, whereby patients 'think by acting upon the psychoanalyst . . . using the analyst's mind as a medium for free-associative thinking' (Bollas 2002: 23). Object relations theory also shows how people can be thought of as having different parts, such as an infant self or an adolescent self, as well as aspects that form around various identifications with significant others, such as parents and siblings. These parts or selves may exist in complex relations to each other, involving internal 'dialogues' that may also be revealed through free association (Bollas 2002: 24–25).

Character too is seen by Bollas as a type of free association in that it 'bears assumptions about being and relating which cannot be thought about at first, but which are always divulged through the idiom of self-expression' (Bollas 2002: 27). Bollas sums up his view as follows:

> Free associating manifests the unconscious. It functions as an ever-sophisticated pathway for the articulation of unconscious ideas, regardless of their derivation: the logic of sequence; the logic of projection; the theatre of parts of the self talking to one another and to parental objects; or the movement of character. (Bollas 2002: 33)

Each of these pathways is relevant in supervision and to the work in supervision of trying to think and talk about what was previously unconscious in the patient. Having explored the concept and method of free association as it was introduced by Freud, and in terms of how it has been used and developed in psychoanalytic thinking since, I am now going to consider free association in relation to supervision.

THE PLACE OF FREE ASSOCIATING IN THE SUPERVISORY RELATIONSHIP

A central function of the supervision of therapy is to facilitate and enable thinking about the supervisee's practice, both with particular patients and more broadly in terms of their overall approach to their work. Presenting work in supervision will always involve exposure and anxiety, and the risk of feeling shame, or even humiliation, as a consequence of that exposure. As such, a supervisor needs to try and create a supervisory space in which there can be a working alliance between supervisor and supervisee that includes feelings of trust and safety. As Mollon says, the 'task [in supervision] is to think and talk freely, reflectively, without censorship, about an experience' (Mollon 1997: 31), and this view of supervision certainly seems congruent with the practice of free association.

Searles writes about the beginning student of therapy in a similar way:

> *Early in supervision, the student often needs to realize that it is all right for him to let his thoughts stray, for example during minutes of silence, away from the patient; he needs to realize, in fact, that a maximal degree of inner freedom to think, fantasy, and feel, is essential to the exercise of his intuition, for unless he can achieve such an inner freedom from his compulsion to help the suffering patient, he will be unable to achieve sufficient distance to note, for example, significant sequences in the patient's associations.* (Searles 1962: 588)

Gee is interested in the supervisor's capacity to associate to material and suggests that an attitude of evenly suspended attention, as recommended by Freud, is appropriate for the supervisor as well as the analyst and can contribute to the development of the supervisee (Gee 1996: 540). He writes:

> *I have found it helpful to 'ponder' aloud on the material that the supervisee brings; in this way the supervisor can encourage the supervisee to 'ponder' on the material. By 'ponder', I mean allowing oneself to consider the possible meaning and purpose of the material in a relatively non-directive way, allowing the material to 'sink-in' while waiting for a thought/feeling/image/insight to arise out of one.* (Gee 1996: 540)

Stewart also sees a place for free association in supervision but at the same time points out that the work with the patient must remain in focus, 'lest associations drift into the realms of private fantasy' (Stewart 2002: 80). He develops this point as follows:

> *The patient's associations are a primary source of information, those of the supervisee may provide access to the countertransference, and the supervisor's associations may also be an informative source of understanding. A supervisor's task is to encourage the supervisees to develop a capacity to associate, so that they can learn to suspend logic and allow the unconscious to 'speak'.* (Stewart 2002: 80)

Here, Stewart seems to envisage the supervisor and supervisee as engaged in a task that is similar to that of the therapist and patient, as described by Bollas: it involves an expansion of the capacity to associate, thereby broadening and perhaps deepening the reach of the unconscious mind of all participants. In this way, supervision can be seen as having a therapeutic potential for both supervisee and supervisor (Driver 2002a: 9).

In supervision where there is room for this kind of associative way of working, whether it be one-to-one or in a group, a situation is created in which insights can arise as part of a process and not necessarily from the person who is the most experienced, in a way that can feel collaborative, perhaps involving a form of play.

Bollas writes that the 'method of free association subverts the psychoanalyst's natural authoritarian tendencies as well as the patient's wish to be dominated by the other's knowledge' (Bollas 2002: 37). I understand him to be talking of how patients can sometimes seem to want to be told what to do or think by their therapists, and how therapists can sometimes find it hard to bear not being directive. I think that his remark can be meaningfully applied to supervision by replacing 'psychoanalyst' with 'supervisor' and 'patient' with 'supervisee'. The supervisor will usually be the more experienced person in the supervisory couple or group and may often have considerable authority invested in him or her, but it is important for supervisors, as well as therapists, to keep in mind that they do not have a monopoly on insight. Furthermore, the fact that there is a process involved in reaching understanding and insight in supervision suggests that any understandings that are arrived at should be regarded as provisional, and fits with the Freudian idea that the patient's material will not necessarily be understood in the here and now, by either supervisee or supervisor.

Thinking about authority, status and power in supervision brings to mind the importance of the transference within the supervisory relationship. A supervisor, like a therapist, needs to be mindful of the transference and countertransference dynamics in their work, and in supervision these can exist between supervisor and supervisee, and supervisor and patient, as well as between supervisee (therapist) and patient. It is clear that in supervision the supervisor will be exposed to the material and impact of the patient through the supervisee's presentation of their work. At the same time, the supervisor is also exposed to the personality of the supervisee to a degree. The supervisor's greater psychological distance from the patient (Searles 1955: 587) may help him or her to take a more objective view of what the patient brings to their therapy, but the supervisor also needs to be alert to the possibility of the supervisee having an impact in supervision that is related to his or her direct experience of the patient and which can happen non-verbally, through projection or projective identification, or what Bollas calls the 'logic of projection'.

It was Searles (1955) who first wrote about what he calls the 'reflection process' in supervision, where difficulties originating in the therapist-patient relationship are unconsciously 'reflected' in the relationship between supervisor and supervisee (therapist). Here too, the supervisor's position of greater distance from the patient may give him or her a better chance of registering something unusual or particular in the supervision, which could be the result of a reflection process, thinking about it, and then being able to put it into words, all of which is a form of associative process that makes use of the supervisor's mind. It is as if there is a train of association that originates in the patient, which may only be articulated initially by the supervisor as a consequence of the emotional impact of the supervisee's presentation.

As I have said, Garland draws our attention to an Oedipal dimension in free association that is to do with being able to allow objects to 'associate freely' with each other (Garland 2002: 508). This idea connects well with existing discussions in the literature on supervision, which examine the three-person nature of the relations in supervision, and the Oedipal dynamics that may follow from this (see for example Driver and Martin 2002; Mander 1993; Mattinson 1981). Supervisees have to be able to tolerate letting supervisors know about their working relationships with patients and what goes on in their consulting rooms. Supervisors have to be able to accept that it is the supervisee who is working with the patient and that supervisees grow and develop and may outgrow their supervisors, just as the relationship between parents and children is always liable to change over time. In addition, both supervisor and supervisee need to have some capacity to tolerate each other associating freely with other objects in their professional lives, such as therapists, teachers and colleagues, as well as with their own minds and thoughts. This last involves the potential for each to arrive at insights and be creative in their work. All of this is part of what can make supervision difficult, complex and emotionally charged but also interesting, satisfying and effective. For Bollas, analytic work that includes free association may extend the realm of what can be thought and said, while, for Garland, it may enhance an individual's capacity to associate freely in relationships. I would want to say that supervision which gives room to free association may be similarly effective in facilitating the development of the supervisee and also of the supervisor and, through their joint efforts, can help develop the therapeutic work with, and for the benefit of, the patient.

Bollas describes free association within the analytic setting as 'the process of speaking oneself in the presence of the other' (Bollas 2002: 63). This is the position of the patient, but in supervision the supervisee is speaking of their work with the patient. While it is clear that one can associate to particular subjects or themes, perhaps there is a question to be asked about whether, or how much, one can associate to the life and experience of someone else without distorting it through the filter of one's own personality and subjectivity.

I think I would want to try and answer this by drawing attention to the fact that the therapist working with the patient has an emotional experience which affects him or her in various ways, both consciously and unconsciously. In supervision, the therapist may be primarily reporting the content and dynamics of their experience of working with the patient, but this can only happen through their awareness, both conscious and unconscious, of their own emotional life and in relation to what in them has been touched by the experience of the other. In other words, there is an important sense in which the supervisee is also 'speaking him, or her, self', talking of their response, their registration, of the patient and of what the patient's impact means to them. However, this does not mean that the supervisee's personality takes centre stage in supervision, as the patient's would, or should, in therapy. The focus in supervision needs to remain on the patient and on the therapist's work with the patient.

In a similar way, the supervisor's attention to their response to the supervisee's presentation could also be seen as an articulation of the supervisor's self within the context of a disciplined professionalism; the aim is not to create a forum for private fantasy but rather to remain attentive to the needs of the patient and to be mindful of the complexity of the supervisory situation. There is distance from the patient as already discussed, but there are also threads of emotional connection at conscious and unconscious levels, and these provide pathways for association that can be fruitful in the understanding of the patient and his or her relationships, both in their inner world and in external reality. In both individual and group supervision, these elements can come into play in a creative way as supervisor and supervisees may each contribute thoughts that help develop the understanding of the patient being presented.

CONSIDERING THE LIMITS TO FREE ASSOCIATION IN SUPERVISION

I have been arguing for the importance of making room for free association in supervision, both on the part of the supervisee and the supervisor. However, it does seem to me that, while free association and associative thinking are necessary within the supervisory situation, they alone are not sufficient to describe an effective methodology of supervision or to preserve good practice. Among other things, there has to be attention to the frame, to boundaries, to the requirements of ethical practice and to all the issues that can arise in relation to each of these, such as the beginnings and endings of sessions, and dealing with the fee in settings where there is one. In this way, supervision is like therapy, since with therapy, too, free association is necessary, but not sufficient, for good practice.

Jacobs et al. (1995) point out that it is important to be respectful of the supervisee's privacy so that explorations of their fantasies and feelings in relation to their work with their patient need to be limited to what is pedagogically useful, thereby maintaining a boundary between supervision and therapy. In their view, the 'use of associative thinking in supervision should not lead to excessive self-exposure on the part of the student', and it 'can be helpful as long as it is within the framework of the educational goal to understand the patient and teach the therapist' (Jacobs et al. 1995: 90).

Another potential limit on free association in supervision arises in relation to clinical responsibility. In some situations, supervisors have a formal responsibility in this area, while in others where they do not they are still likely to feel a concern for the patient's welfare. In this context, the supervisor may sometimes feel a need to ask direct questions or seek particular information in order to clarify the circumstances of the patient's current life situation. It is rather like being in the position of a passenger in Freud's imaginary train carriage, who, unable to see out of the window, asks a fellow passenger for a description of the view or seeks further information about some of what has been described. For example, if a supervisor were concerned about a patient's depression getting worse, he or she might need to know whether the therapist thought that the patient was suicidal, whether the patient had seen their doctor or whether the therapist had discussed with the patient the possibility of going to see their doctor.

Supervisors may have other responsibilities, such as that of assessing a trainee's progress within a training organization. Here, the supervisory relationship will be affected by the requirement for assessment, and this is likely to increase the supervisee's anxiety, who may then find it more difficult to talk freely for fear of exposing mistakes, of getting it wrong or of getting a bad assessment. The supervisor of trainees is also likely to be the subject of transferences in a more general way that may have an inhibiting effect on the trainee's ability to associate, depending on what the prevailing view of the supervisor is and on the particular dynamics of the supervisory relationship.

If the supervisor notices a decrease in associative thinking on the part of the supervisee, this could in itself be a useful indication of increased anxiety, which could then be discussed with the supervisee in an attempt to free up the supervisory space. On the other hand, it should also be borne in mind that a decrease in associative thinking could also be due to the patient's state of mind, creating an atmosphere in which thought is restricted. In general, one would usually expect trainees to become more able to associate to their experience of the patient the further on they are within their training, particularly when the training is one that requires the trainee to be in therapy. In other words, the trainee's capacity to associate might be a consideration in the assessment process itself.

The practice of free association in supervision also raises a question about the use of notes, both by the supervisee and the supervisor. Historically, there have been two schools of thought about supervision in psychoanalytic training, one of which separated the roles of analyst and supervisor while the other had supervision of a training case carried out by the analyst (Martin 2002). In relation to these two schools of thought, it is possible to identify two traditions over notes: where analyst and supervisor were one and the same person, it seems that the clinical work was presented to the supervisor/analyst through the means of free association, without any notes, and with the trainee perhaps lying on the couch. This at least was the experience of Michael Balint, as reported by Pedder (Pedder 1986: 7). Where the roles of analyst and supervisor were carried out by different people, the trainee might still have presented their work through free association, but, in fact, a tradition of providing written reports of sessions has developed, and is now widely practised in the supervision of counselling and therapy.

In my own work as a supervisor, I ask supervisees to bring notes in the form of a process report that gives a sense of the flow of the session: who said what, when and what was the response? Sometimes notes can be used defensively, so that supervision can become filled by the report of a session, but it is my experience overall that having the supervisee use notes does not preclude free association. In some ways, I think that a supervisee's verbatim report of a session is something of a useful fiction: it can never fully capture the session as it was, but it can give some idea of how the supervisee experiences and processes a session, and it can also of itself provide a basis for free associating, both in the writing of it and in the presenting of it in supervision, when the supervisor can create space for more spontaneous reflection and talking by encouraging the supervisee to put their notes aside, as it were, some of the time.

When working in organizational settings, supervisors are likely to be expected, or required, to keep some record of what is happening in the therapeutic work, and my own preference when working in private practice is also to take notes. However, I find that my approach to taking notes is far from systematic and moves between different intentions: sometimes I try to take an accurate and fairly detailed record of a session, and this is usually if I am concerned about the patient, the work being done or struggling to follow the material. At other times, I may only be noting a few words or phrases that for some reason catch my attention in a particular way. In this latter case, it seems to me that there is a preconscious or unconscious resonance generated by the material, and the note I make allows me to return to what was said and try to understand its meaning. A problem with taking notes is that it does interfere with being in a state of evenly suspended attention, but, on the other hand, the notes I take can in themselves provide a prompt for useful associative work, and I think that this supervisory aim, of fostering free association, needs to be kept in mind alongside whatever requirement for records there may be.

CONCLUSION

Although Freud never wrote about supervision as such, one could say that in the case history of Little Hans, he is essentially in the position of a supervisor, hearing about the case material from one of his 'adherents' (Freud 1909: 170), who is also Hans' father. Since Freud's account of the case was published, psychoanalytic theory and practice have developed enormously, and, as part of that development, supervision has emerged as a specialism in its own right, while the method of free association has remained central to psychoanalytic work.

The supervisory relationship is one of richness and complexity, which requires the supervisor to be able to listen and respond to the supervisee's presentation from a number of different perspectives and 'to be both inside and outside the supervisory relationship, that is to be both subjective and objective' (Driver 2002b: 55). In this chapter, I have put forward a case for the importance of making room for free association in supervision, for both supervisee and supervisor, while acknowledging that free association is not in itself sufficient for the safe practice of supervision. A benefit of this position is that it establishes common ground between working as a therapist and working as a supervisor, while at the same time allowing for the differences between these activities.

REFERENCES

Bellow S (2001) Ravelstein. London: Penguin Books.

Bollas C (2002) Free Association. Cambridge: Icon Books.

Bronstein C (2002) On free association and psychic reality. British Journal of Psychotherapy 18(4): 477–489.

Driver C (2002a) 'Introduction: orientation and themes'. In Driver C, Martin E (eds) (2002) Supervising Psychotherapy. London: Sage Publications.

Driver C (2002b) 'Internal states in the supervisory relationship'. In Driver C, Martin E (eds), Supervising Psychotherapy. London: Sage Publications.

Driver C, Martin E (eds) (2002) Supervising Psychotherapy. London: Sage Publications.

Freud A (1936) The Ego and the Mechanisms of Defence. London: Hogarth Press.

Freud S (1909) Analysis of a Phobia in a Five-year-old Boy ('Little Hans'). Penguin Freud Library 8. London: Penguin Books.

Freud S (1912) Recommendations to Physicians Practising Psycho-Analysis. SE 12. London: Hogarth Press.

Freud S (1913) On Beginning the Treatment. SE 12. London: Hogarth Press.

Freud S (1923) Two Encyclopaedia Articles. Penguin Freud Library 15. London: Penguin Books.

Freud S (1925) An Autobiographical Study. Penguin Freud Library 15. London: Penguin Books.

Freud S, Breuer J (1895) Studies on Hysteria. Penguin Freud Library 3. London: Penguin Books.

Garland C (2002) The open mind and some of its anxieties. British Journal of Psychotherapy. 18(4): 491–508.

Gee H (1996) Developing insight through supervision: relating, then defining. Journal of Analytical Psychology 41(4): 529–552.

Jacobs D, David P, Meyer DJ (1995) The Supervisory Encounter. New Haven and London: Yale University Press.

Kris A (1996) Free Association: Method and Process (revised edition). London: Karnac Books.

Laplanche J, Pontalis JB (1973) The Language of Psycho-Analysis. London: Hogarth Press.

Mander G (1993) Dyads and triads: some thoughts on the nature of therapy supervision. Journal of the Institute of Psychotherapy and Counselling 1: 1–10.

Martin E (2002) 'Listening to the absent patient: therapeutic aspects of supervision'. In Driver C, Martin E (eds), Supervising Psychotherapy. London: Sage Publications.

Mattinson J (1981) The Deadly Equal Triangle. Northampton, MA and London: The Smith College School of Social Work and the Group of the Advancement of Psychotherapy in Social Work.

Mawson C (2002) Pseudo-free association: the sophisticated analytic patient and 'as-if' relating. British Journal of Psychotherapy 18(4): 509–522.

Mitchell SA, Black MJ (1995) Freud and Beyond. New York: Basic Books.

Mollon P (1997) 'Supervision as a space for thinking'. In Shipton G (ed.), Supervision of Psychotherapy and Counselling: Making a Place to Think. Buckingham: Open University Press.

Pedder J (1986) Reflections on the theory and practice of supervision. Psychoanalytic Psychotherapy 2(1): 1–12.

Searles H (1955) 'The informational value of the supervisor's emotional experiences'. In Searles H (1965) Collected Papers on Schizophrenia and Related Subjects. London: Hogarth Press.

Searles H (1962) 'Problems of psycho-analytic supervision'. In Searles H (1965) Collected Papers on Schizophrenia and Related Subjects. London: Hogarth Press.

Stewart J (2002) 'The interface between teaching and supervision'. In Driver C, Martin E (eds), Supervising Psychotherapy. London: Sage Publications..

Williams P (2002) Un-free associations: introductory remarks. British Journal of Psychotherapy 18(4): 471–476.

Winnicott DW (1985a) Playing and Reality. Harmondsworth: Penguin Books. First published in 1971.

Winnicott DW (1985b) 'Playing: creative activity and the search for the self'. In Winnicott DW (1985a), Playing and Reality. Harmondsworth: Penguin Books.

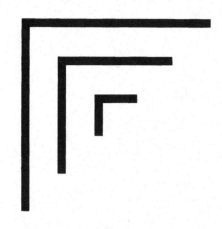

THE SUPERVISORY RELATIONSHIP

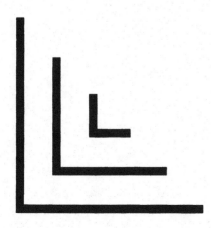

CHAPTER 5

ATTACHMENT AND THE SUPERVISORY ALLIANCE

CHRISTINE DRIVER

INTRODUCTION

Supervision has, as its aim, the purpose of creating meaning out of the narrative that the patient brings as well as understanding the manifestation of the patient's inner-world struggles as they are expressed through their interaction and relationship with the therapist. Interaction and relationship with the therapist generates relational dynamics that will be affected by the inner-world assumptions of each person. Indeed, an understanding and awareness of how an alliance is formed in a relationship will need to take these relational dynamics into account. Attachment theory and recent explorations into attachment, internal working models, narrative competence and reflective function have something important to contribute to developmental and psychoanalytic theories. Consideration of attachment issues, and attachment-based research in relation to therapy, is developing rapidly, and clearly a chapter on such a vast subject cannot hope to do it justice. However, what is becoming increasingly apparent is that the ideas and discoveries that are emerging have something important to contribute in understanding relationships, especially those in which vulnerability, dependency and attachment play a part. Clinical supervision is one such relationship.

ATTACHMENT AND THE INTERNAL WORKING MODEL

Since the original work by Bowlby (1981) into attachment, there has been considerable study and research by such people as Ainsworth et al. (1978), Bretherton (1991), Bretherton and Munholland (1999), Holmes (2002), Fonagy

(2001), Main (1991), Knox (2003), Diamond and Marrone (2003), Cortina and Marrone (2003) and others into the implications of maternal attunement and attachment. Ainsworth (Holmes 2002: 105), in her studies, identifies four major attachment patterns in relation to attachment and separation. She defines these patterns of attachment as secure, insecure, insecure ambivalent and insecure disorganized. The importance of these attachment patterns with the original caregiver are that they influence and determine the development of internal working models (Holmes 2002: 76), mentalization and reflective function (Fonagy and Target 1998: 91).

Studies (Bretherton cited in Holmes 2002: 122) reveal that internal working models reflect an internal organization of mental functioning that has developed in relation to attachment experience and adaptation. It is significant, and something borne out by studies of narrative capacities, that the infant's experience of attachment (or failure thereof) and maternal attunement will influence mental functioning. As Diamond and Marrone comment, 'Parent–child interactional patterns become internal structures (internal working models) with organising functions over the psychological, psychosomatic and psychosocial life of the individual' (Diamond and Marrone 2003: 5).

The significance of the findings of this research for the 'relational' therapies is that internal working models will affect, and influence, the dynamic of the relationship. Internal working models 'store accumulated experience of early relationships into patterns of meaning which determine a person's attitude and behaviour in subsequent relationships' (Knox 2003: 54) and influence the ability to relate to and understand 'the psychological characteristics of other people' (Fonagy 2001: 14). This clearly has important implications in work, such as supervision, in which part of the process is to understand the other, the patient.

ATTACHMENT AND THE THERAPEUTIC AND SUPERVISORY PARADIGM

The implications of attachment theory in relation to psychotherapy are beginning to be explored, and Holmes (2002: 149) considers how the 'core attachment status' of an individual will affect and influence their relational behaviour. He comments, 'where there is a secure core state, a person feels good about themselves and their capacity to be effective and pursue their projects. Where the core state is insecure, defensive strategies come into play' (Holmes 2002: 149). Holmes, in his exploration, considers the way in which attachment issues influence interpersonal relationships and interpersonal defences and the manner in which a person creates a narrative about their history. He goes on to look at how the core attachment status influences the establishment of the therapeutic relationship, the therapeutic alliance, the autobiographical competence of the patient, the ability of the patient to process affect and to reflect on, and integrate, experience, and he examines these issues in relation to therapy. Holmes (2002) cites Frank's 'common factors' in therapy and 'the key elements which are shared by all therapies. These include a *relationship* with the therapist . . . in Bowlbian terms a secure base from which to start to explore the problem: a coherent *explanation* for the patient's difficulties – a shared narrative and a *method* for overcoming them' (Holmes 2002: 151). These 'key elements' of relationship, explanation and method also play an important role in supervision, and clearly issues of attachment, in relation to clinical and supervisory work, cannot be overlooked.

More recently, issues of attachment and the influence of internal working models in relation to the therapeutic relationship and transference dynamics have been explored further. Diamond et al. report that 'patients' internal working models of attachment affect a number of aspects of the therapeutic endeavour, including (1) the nature of the patient's symptom reporting, (2) the capacity to make use of treatment, (3) the quality of the therapeutic alliance, and (4) treatment outcome' (Diamond et al. 2003: 132). However, the therapeutic endeavour, and the understanding of the patient and their inner world, doesn't just occur in the consulting room; it also, and significantly, occurs within supervision. Indeed, supervision, and especially within a training, is a relationship that is specifically geared for the purpose of understanding another, the patient. Within the supervisory relationship, alliance and attachment are important and attachment patterns and internal working models will inevitably influence the way that supervisor and supervisee attach, interact, develop a narrative and empathically and reflectively understand and gain insight about the patient.

The exploratory process in supervision therefore requires that both supervisor and supervisee develop a variety of modes of functioning. It requires the formation of an alliance in relation to the 'absent patient' (Martin 2002), the development of internal mental functioning and reflection in relation to the development of the 'internal supervisor' (Casement 1985), the ability to think about thinking, and the generation of processes of understanding, appraisal, meaning and learning in relation to the patient. Each of these processes requires an interrelational dynamic both interpersonally and intrapsychically.

The development of the 'internal supervisor', as envisaged by Casement (1985), occurs through stages of engagement with, and internalization of, the external supervisor, culminating in the integration of the 'supervisor' into an aspect of the self. The functioning of the internal supervisor is dependent upon the development of the ability to observe and think about the processes occurring within oneself, that is to develop the capacity to reflect on, think about and process what you are thinking or feeling, such that experience is experienced, observed and thought about more or less simultaneously. This ability to twin-track intrapsychically, and within the interactive processes between supervisor, supervisee and patient, allows both subjective and objective experience to be thought about and processed. Such a process requires the development of the reflective function to appraise, process and make sense of the narrative and the experience. It is within these processes of observation, reflection, appraisal and thought that the information emerges about what is self and what is other, that is what belongs to me and what belongs to the patient.

These processes of observation, reflection and thought require the supervisee to make both assimilative and accommodative (see Chapter 2's footnote: 19) shifts that combine emotional and cognitive processes in order to identify, think about and make conscious the mental and emotional patterns of the internal world of the patient. Diamond and Marrone identify a similar point when they cite Stern, who describes 'how therapeutic shifts come about not through any act of cognition but are to do with an affective understanding implicit in intersubjective moments, that is the way of being together of analyst and analysand. These give rise to a reorganization of the analysand's way of being with others, his "implicit relational knowing"' (Diamond and Marrone 2003: 146). In a similar way, true understanding of the patient by the supervisee comes via 'affective understanding'. This may involve links to theoretical constructs, but it also requires an interplay within the supervisory alliance between the thinking and reflective functions of both supervisee and supervisor. The ability to generate an 'affective understanding' of the patient will be affected by the professional and personal developmental status of the supervisee, the degree to which anxiety dominates, the internal working model of the supervisee and their ability to form an alliance and attachment to a process in which they can think about the other, the patient.

ATTACHMENT AND THE SUPERVISORY ALLIANCE

The supervisory relationship is one that requires a working alliance between both parties (supervisor and supervisee) and requires an engagement with conscious and unconscious processes in order to understand the patient through the narrative that the supervisee brings. The influence of attachment patterns in supervision is one that Bowlby considers, and he 'noted that in supervision . . . those preoccupied with attachment issues *were* inhibited in their thinking and in explorative reflection' (Diamond and Marrone 2003: 148). Given that supervision is always a relationship in which vulnerability plays some part, attachment dynamics will frequently be activated when a supervisee comes for supervision, especially if the supervisee is new to counselling or psychotherapy or is attending supervision within the context of a training. As Liotti (1999) comments, 'It should be remembered, moreover, that expressing one's vulnerability and sufferings in dialogue with a person that comes to be perceived as stronger and/or wiser than the self – as is the case of the patient in the thera-peutic relationship – leads to the activation of the attachment system' (Liotti 1999: 769). Just as this is true for a patient attending therapy, it is equally true for new supervisees attending supervision within a training setting in which the relationship is influenced by anxiety, vulnerability, dependence, appraisal and an asymmetric balance of power.

In supervision, the supervisee, especially at the start of training, often feels far from secure, and this activates attachment and defensive proclivities in rela-tion to real or imagined anxieties and vulnerabilities. The following conversation might be overheard in many settings: 'What's your new supervi-sor like? Is she demanding? Do you get on with her?' The colleague replies, 'Well she's all right. She challenged me a lot, but she made me think. I learnt a lot.' The first supervisee replies, 'Well, I'm glad I'm not with her; I don't think I'd get on with her and she makes me anxious. I'd just clam up.' This snippet of conversation reflects the way that many supervisees weigh up how they would get on with a supervisor and reflects how supervisees frequently assess how well they will attach to the supervisor and, by implication, what they feel they would learn from supervision.

The personal issues and learning needs that a supervisee new to counselling and psychotherapy work brings to supervision are explored by Stoltenberg and Delworth. They point out that a new, Level 1, trainee is dependent on the super-visor, highly motivated, imitative, anxious and that they are 'neurosis bound, lacking self-awareness and other-awareness' (Stoltenberg and Delworth 1987: 52). Similarly, Hawkins and Shohet comment that the focus of a new supervisee is primarily self-centred and that they often come with the question 'Can I make it in this work?' (Hawkins and Shohet 2002: 64). The dependency needs of a new supervisee not only relate to the need to learn and develop understanding about clinical work but also relate to their need for a secure space in which they can feel supported in that exploration. However, they also bring with them their own internal working models of relationship and attachment assumptions, and in this beginning phase these can tend to dominate the patient's material.

> This was evident when supervisee Dee, in her presentation of patient C, interspersed her description of the session with comments like 'but life isn't like that', 'surely people don't behave in that way' and 'can't she [patient C] see that if she's always aggressive people won't like her?' Although these comments reflected transference issues for the patient, it was evident, at the time, that they reflected the way that the supervisee was imposing her views onto the clinical material. In this early phase of the clinical work, Dee's focus was largely self-centred; she lacked the ability to empathize with different situations and to consider and reflect on internal working models different to her own.

The example illustrates how internal working models and attachment issues affect the clinical relationship. As Pistole and Watkins comment, 'The pattern of attachment is also relevant because beliefs about the self and other, as well as strategies that regulate affect and attention to attachment information, guide behavior in important relationships' (Pistole and Watkins 1995: 459). The above example reflects this and illustrates how the supervisee remained caught within her own perspective. This perspective tended towards concrete and presymbolic thinking, and Dee did not yet have the capacity to contain the experience of the patient and reflect and think about the patient's communication and internal world as something separate and different from her own.

Watkins (1995) has made a particular study of attachment styles in relation to supervision and the supervisory alliance. He considers how attachment styles, such as anxious or ambivalent attachment, compulsive self-reliance and compulsive caregiving, affect supervision. In his explorations, Watkins cites an example of the difficulty of supervising a supervisee whose attachment style was of compulsive self-reliance and demonstrates how this impeded the supervisory alliance, reflective processes and learning within supervision. Watkins is clear in his view that pathologically attached supervisees need to be in psychotherapy not supervision and that supervision is not the forum for 'treatment' because, as he comments, 'we risk patient care to accommodate supervisee pathology' (Watkins 1995: 338). This is certainly the case where supervisee attachment styles impede the supervisory relationship, learning, reflection and processing.

Watkins tends to focus on the behaviour of the supervisee in relation to a specific attachment pattern and is very negative about the outcome, concluding that certain attachment styles are not conducive to clinical working and learning within supervision. Although Watkins' view is somewhat pessimistic and tends to exclude the impact of the supervisee's therapy, when it occurs simultaneously to training, he is raising a very important issue. What Watkins identifies is that unless attachment patterns are considered in relation to supervision and the supervisory alliance their impact on the supervisory process and the development of learning, reflection and understanding are overlooked. Supervision, and the supervisory alliance, depends on processes of cooperation and co-thinking to develop an understanding of the patient, their unconscious communications and the development of the clinical work. Attachment patterns and internal working models will inevitably impact on this and will affect and influence the dynamic.

Diamond et al. also present some very interesting findings from their research into attachment issues and therapy and present an example (Diamond et al. 2003: 164) of how the therapist's attachment style affected, and conflated with, the transference and attachment dynamic from the patient. The research that they have carried out demonstrates the importance of attachment issues in relation to the therapeutic alliance and the therapeutic dynamic, but they caution that the 'causal relationship is not simple or linear but rather the result of goodness of fit between the individual's inner organization and the multifaceted contexts in which it evolves' (Diamond et al. 2003: 171). What this would seem to indicate is that when there is a willingness to engage in a process by both parties, that is supervisor and supervisee, there is an engagement with the dynamic, which can encourage a supervisory alliance and processes of 'co-thinking' (Diamond and Marrone 2003: 125), co-reflection and 'bloody serious play' (Szecsödy 1997: 113) between supervisor and supervisee and generate accommodative learning and internal shifts.

Holmes (2002) identifies three fundamental elements that make a secure base in therapy. These are 'attunement, the fostering of autobiographical competence and affective processing' (Holmes 2002: 155-156), and he explores the issues of attachment and internal working models in relation to the therapeutic milieu and the therapeutic alliance. Within supervision, the supervisory alliance also needs to provide a secure base in which there is attunement between supervisor and supervisee in relation to the patient's material, narrative competence in relation to the patient's conscious and unconscious communications and affective processing in relation to the patient's narrative and unconscious communications within the transference and countertransference. In many respects, aspects of supervision parallel, and link to, attachment issues and internal working models as identified within the therapeutic frame. This is because the supervisory relationship is also one in which an external and internal alliance is required so that the dynamics of the process, and the internal world issues and internal working model of the patient, can be explored, processed and reflected on.

THE SUPERVISORY ALLIANCE AND INTERNAL WORKING MODELS

In relation to how we work as supervisors, it is important to consider how attachment issues, and the internal working model of the supervisee (and supervisor), affect the therapeutic work and the supervisory relationship. This is not to say that the boundary between supervision and therapy is to be breached but seen rather as a way of understanding aspects of the complex dynamics of the supervisory relationship and the learning needs of the supervisee. The impact of internal working models and attachment patterns can have a powerful influence on the dynamic with the patient and the supervisor, as the following example illustrates.

A supervisee, Sue, had been allocated to a supervisor within a training set-ting. Sue had been seeing patients for about a year but had had difficulty in holding and sustaining work with them. When she started in supervision, she had one patient who she had been seeing for about nine months. In the initial supervisory session, she expressed her anxiety about talking about this patient to a new supervisor because she feared that 'new input' would upset the relationship with the patient, and she feared she would lose her.

The supervisor was aware of Sue's anxiety and decided not to chal-lenge her at this point. As the supervision progressed, however, it became apparent that Sue was highly ambivalent towards supervision. There was a resistance to hearing the supervisor's input and reflections, and Sue tended to operate from the defensive position in which she deemed her view of her patients to be right. The fact that she exhibited this rela-tionship to the supervisor in relation to all her subsequent patients made the supervisor aware that this was not an aspect of the reflection process, in relation to unconscious communications from a particular patient, but was intrinsic to Sue and her relationship patterns.

The supervisory relationship with Sue was therefore coloured throughout by her attachment style and her internal working model. Sue was ambivalent and tended to operate from a position of compul-sive self-reliance. This made it difficult for a supervisory relationship to develop and, as a result, difficult for her to develop a reflective function in relation to the patient's material, especially in relation to the impact of the patient's transferences and unconscious communication.

In terms of the supervisory alliance, it is important that a secure and trust-ing attachment and engagement between supervisor and supervisee develops for such an alliance to be generated. It is within this alliance that a process of exploration and reflection, which mirrors and embodies that of the reflective function that Fonagy (2001) refers to, can occur. It is through the supervisor's reflective, cognitive and empathic engagement with the supervisee and the patient that understanding can develop from the conscious and unconscious narratives of the supervisee and the patient. A working supervisory alliance enables engagement with, and exploration and appraisal of, the patient's mate-rial in a manner that facilitates the supervisee to generate the development of their own reflective function. Casement (1985) refers to this process but under somewhat different terms in relation to the internal supervisor. But the paral-lels with attachment theory allow us to consider wider dynamics in relation to the supervisory relationship and the supervisory alliance and to consider how we work with the impact of internal working models on the supervisory relationship. We return to the example with Sue.

It became apparent to the supervisor that Sue's pattern of relating, and her transference to the supervisor, generated an attachment style in which learning could not take place. For Sue, the supervisor's reflections about her patient's communication were experienced as criticism rather than additional information based on the patient's communication. Sue's narrative about her patient, and the material that the patient presented, was frequently based on perceptions based on Sue's internal working models, and she was unable to accommodate and assimilate those of others when considering her patient. It became evident through the supervision that, just as she couldn't 'hear' the supervisor, Sue could not 'hear' what her patient was saying and tended to make interpretations to the patient based on her own internal working models. When, however, this patient subsequently left, Sue and the supervisor were, at last, able to begin to consider the difficulty of hearing and understanding the mind of another, whether that was the patient or the supervisor.

A positive aspect of this, however, was that Sue was aware she could not learn from the supervisor and that she was being defensive about her work and was able to pursue this in her own therapy. The supervisor was also aware that there was a joint dynamic between Sue and herself and that her 'attachment style' had, initially, fuelled Sue's defensive withdrawal. The supervisor realized, on reflection, that she had initially seen Sue as withdrawn and had got drawn into a critical engagement to try to elicit a response. However, inevitably, the response it evoked was further anxious and defensive withdrawal by Sue.

This potential to create a vicious circle of attachment and transference dynamics is a dilemma that a supervisor has to consider, especially when there is a breakdown in the supervisory relationship. Stimmel (1995) considers the issue of the supervisor's countertransference, and this is surely a factor in any supervisory relationship. Within a training setting this is a powerful dynamic because the supervisor holds the power over whether the supervisee 'passes or fails'. It is when there are difficulties in the supervisor–supervisee relationship that issues such as attachment status and transference are important factors to consider. Supervisors sometimes describe an impasse in supervision as a 'personality clash', or a 'breakdown in communication' when what they may also be describing is a clash of attachment patterns, attunement, internal working models and the way that meaning is derived from experience. It is important, therefore, that the supervisor is aware of the power of these attachment dynamics and of how the supervisor's own attachment style can generate resistant and defensive dynamics within the supervisee.

In terms of the supervisor–supervisee relationship the place for explorations of these personal issues is within personal exploration and therapy. However, supervision can also mediate their influence through being holding and non-retaliatory such that it mediates the assumptions that the supervisee brings. This is problematic, however, when there is concern in relation to the professional competence of the supervisee and the way this is reflected in their inability to learn from and make use of supervision. Here, the supervisor may have no other choice but to confront and appraise the supervisee in relation to a lack of clinical or ethical competence.

Attachment patterns between supervisor and supervisee clearly impact on the supervisory alliance, and personal dynamics are important factors in relation to the development of a supervisory and learning alliance. Initially, internal working models may dominate because the supervisory relationship encompasses dependency needs along with anxieties about 'survival', and internal working models of ambivalence, self-reliance, disorganization etc. will almost inevitably be evident at the early stages of supervision. What the supervisor needs to aim for, and provide, is a pattern of relationship in which there is an empathic understanding of the underlying anxiety about being a beginner in which reflection and exploration within a secure environment can be encouraged.

However, the supervisor also holds the aspect of assessment. This dynamic contains the need to balance assessment and appraisal without becoming a persecutory superego figure. The dilemma for the supervisor is that reflection and input will be judged by the internal working models of the supervisee, and the learning and professional development of the supervisee will spiral through (Perry 2003) intrapsychic and interpsychic processes in relation to the self, the patient and the supervisee. Perry relates this process to a three-dimensional matrix in which 'the whole matrix quivers, sending potential resonances of meaning and growth along each and every strand simultaneously' (Perry 2003: 204) and which, for Perry, 'the matrix implies, and has faith in, a developmental (including regressive) and teleological thrust in all the parties concerned' (Perry 2003: 205). Within any significant relationship, there will be resonances, reverberations and impact, at a variety of levels, consciously and unconsciously. Supervision is one such significant relationship within therapeutic work and as such holds an important dynamic in relation to internal working models and the development of the reflective function.

INTERNAL WORKING MODELS AND THE REFLECTIVE FUNCTION

The ability to attach to, relate to and understand the mind of another depends to a large degree on the development of the reflective function. Within a secure attachment, the mother's reflective function will enable the infant to develop that capacity for themselves, which will, in turn, create for the infant a sense of autobiographical self, an ability to create a narrative of experience, and a capacity to have a 'theory of mind' about self and other. Reflective function refers to an 'understanding of feeling states in self and others that is formed through our affective relations with others' (Diamond and Marrone 2003: 146) but is not to be confused with 'introspection or self-consciousness' (Diamond and Marrone 2003: 143). Reflective function is a term, therefore, that incorporates the concepts of 'metacognitive monitoring', 'mind-mindedness' and 'theory of mind' and refers to the development of a reflective capacity in relation to self and other. Knox (2003) identifies four key and interrelated components in relation to the development of reflective function:

> narrative competence: *the recognition of psychological cause and effect, which links events in a meaningful way and is the basis for a sense of agency*
>
> intentionality: *the capacity to pursue goals and desires, that is, to have a mental appetite*
>
> appraisal: *the capacity to evaluate the relative significance of experiences*
>
> individuation: *the awareness of one's own and other people's independent subjectivity*
>
> (Knox 2003: 142)

The aim of supervisee development could be seen, therefore, as a process that enables the supervisee to develop their reflective function in terms of appraisal, narrative competence, intentionality and individuation. In some senses this reflects the development towards the experienced clinician, outlined by Stoltenberg and Delworth, whereby the therapist 'is able to focus intently on the client, empathetically understand his or her world, and still pull back and objectively process information – including his or her own reactions' (Stoltenberg and Delworth 1987: 95).

The ability of the supervisee and supervisor to engage in supervision, however, depends on the supervisee's ability to present a coherent narrative of the content of the sessions with the patient and their reflections on the manner of engagement between patient and therapist. Discussions around taping, verbatims and process recordings of sessions are part of the debate and concern of how the true nature of the session with the patient is reported within supervision. The dilemma, however, is that although taping and verbatims may well recreate the verbal content of the session they do not necessarily reflect what the supervisee has understood and processed in relation to the patient or how the supervisee has understood the patient's narrative in terms of conscious and unconscious content.

Learning processes within supervision, therefore, need to enable the supervisee to develop narrative competence because what the supervisee has been able to 'hear' and conceptualize in relation to the patient will determine what is brought to supervision and the narrative form in which it is presented. Allowing the supervisee to recreate a session in their own words immediately gives an insight as to how the supervisee is relating to the patient's material. The supervisee's own narrative therefore acts as an entry point into both the patient's material and the way that the supervisee has made sense of it.

A supervisee brought notes about a patient session that focused, almost exclusively, on the manifest content of the sessions. The supervisee went on to describe how the patient had talked about various family and work events. These had been told to the therapist in a very factual way, but the supervisor was aware of an undercurrent of anxiety. As the supervisee narrated the content of the session, the manner of her reporting indicated that the supervisee had responded to the patient in a very explanatory way, and the narrative style of the supervisee, in supervision, reflected an impatience and disdain with the infantile nature of the patient's relationship to the world.

As the supervisor reflected internally on the supervisee's presentation, it seemed that the supervisee's anxiety was high, her superego tended to rule her thinking and attitude towards the patient by getting caught into telling her what to do and that an anxious/ambivalent attachment operated in relation to both the patient and the supervisor. In addition, it was apparent that both the patient and the therapist were only able to consider the issues talked about at a superficial and conscious level.

The supervisor explored with the supervisee how the patient described and generated infantile attachments whereby she elicited help and explanations about being 'told what to do' and that this was what the supervisee was presenting in her narrative of the work. It was also apparent from the narrative that the patient's anxiety about 'what she should do' dominated all aspects of her life. These reflections prompted, within the supervisee, processes of appraisal and separation. She was able to see that part of the superego anxiety was her own but that the larger part belonged to the patient. She also realized that just as she had kept the narrative of the session 'superficial and conscious', so the patient kept her narratives of her daily events 'superficial and conscious' in order to avoid being in touch with her internal fears and anxieties, especially about being 'attacked'. In addition, the joint reflection by the supervisor and the supervisee enabled a consideration of the disdain and impatience that was expressed within the narrative of the supervisee.

This appraisal of the narrative, and the unconscious processes caught up in it, enabled a consideration of the transference and the internal working model of the patient. This indicated an ambivalent and anxious attachment, that the patient operated from an infant–like and dependent state but that she also carried an unconscious and internal disdain of the 'infantile'. The consideration of these narrative dynamics enabled an understanding of the patient's internal objects and parental imagos. It was apparent that the internal working model of the patient not only affected the way the patient narrated her experience but also how the therapist responded to the patient and what the therapist brought into supervision in terms of her narrative style.

This exploration by both supervisor and supervisee enabled a reflective process in which both pursued the goal of understanding (intentionality), 'narrative competence' in relation to a recognition of 'psychological cause and effect' (Knox 2003: 142), appraisal of the experience of both self and other, and the development of an understanding of the meaning of the experience of the therapist and the patient, that is an 'awareness of one's own and other people's independent subjectivity' (Knox 2003: 143). The supervisee was therefore able to develop an understanding of what belonged to the patient and what belonged to her, and from this develop a theory about the patient's internal world. She was able to think about her own experience of the patient and understand the dynamics and realize that the patient constantly related to others as an 'insecure child' eliciting parental responses which maintained an infantile dependency. It was through these processes of reflection and appraisal with the supervisor that the supervisee developed her own independent and individuated understanding about the patient.

The kind of reflective exploration outlined above probably forms part of many supervisory encounters. The reflection, exploration and appraisal of the supervisee's narrative and narrative style provide a way of exploring the conscious and unconscious processes and conscious and unconscious communications within the therapeutic and supervisory relationship. What the supervisee brings, what they remember, how they relate to it and the countertransference responses of both supervisee and supervisor are key considerations in the understanding of the patient, as Searles (1955/1986) and Mattinson (1981) amongst others point out. When a supervisor can make use of their reflective function in relation to the clinical material and the supervisory relationship, they model a process with and for the supervisee in relation to these dynamics. If we return to Knox's ideas, it is clearly important for the supervisor to develop their own capacity to remain curious, have 'mental appetite' (Knox 2003: 142) and appraise content, narrative and experience. Equally, it is important that the supervisor has a sense of their own agency and authority and can remain mindful and reflective about themselves and the other in order to work with the supervisee to develop thought and mindfulness about the

patient. It is through these interactive processes with the supervisor that supervisees develop their own capacity to reflect and appraise content, narrative and
experience and develop and individuate as practitioners.

NARRATIVE AND MEMORY

The narrative descriptions of a session that a supervisee brings will, therefore,
inevitably depend on what they remember. Memory is affected by unconscious
processes and reflects what can be held in mind for conscious thought and
what is defended against, forgotten and remains unconscious. The two types of
memory that attachment research has identified (Knox 1999: 513) are declarative memory and implicit memory. Declarative memory refers primarily to the
'conscious retrieval of information about past events and experiences' (Knox
1999: 513), and implicit memory 'stores sequences of actions, general rules
about how things are done . . . *and* stores information about patterns of relationship' (Knox 1999: 514). These implicit memories influence us without our
being consciously aware of them and are 'formed by internalization of the
external world' (Knox 1999: 513).

In a process such as supervision in which memory plays such a vital part, it
is important to be aware of how unconscious processes, defences and implicit
and declarative memory will influence and affect what is remembered of the
conscious narrative of a session and the interactive processes (for example transference, countertransference, projections etc.) with the patient. It is within this
dynamic that aspects of the internal world of the patient will be reflected and
conveyed and affected by the internal working model of the supervisee.

> A supervisee, Dan, presented in supervision a patient who repeatedly
> missed sessions and who often expressed doubts as to how therapy
> could help her. The patient was having difficulties in her relationship
> with her partner and was wondering whether to end the relationship.
> Dan, in his presentations in supervision, was simultaneously dismissive
> of the patient and found it difficult to remember exactly what she had
> been saying about her situation or his interpretations to her. The super-
> visor explored with Dan what the patient's difficulties, and ambivalence
> about the relationship, linked to and of how a parallel level of ambiva-
> lence was being expressed by Dan. Dan commented that he felt the
> patient was dismissive of men and that this riled him, and he could see
> how this caused him to feel ambivalent and dismissive towards her.
> As we explored further, it became apparent how the patient's ambiva-
> lent attachment to a parental figure held an unconscious dismissal
> of men. This unconscious attack on Dan, as therapist, triggered

unconscious and internal issues for him, which in turn affected what he could remember of the session.

Narrative competence requires the ability to talk objectively about experience (Holmes 2002: 9). Holmes goes on to comment, 'Narrative turns experience into a story which is temporal, is coherent and has meaning . . . it creates out of fragmentary experience an unbroken line or thread linking the present with the past and future' (Holmes 2002: 150). Listening to the narrative within therapy is essential for the therapist, but, equally, listening to the narrative and style of that narrative within supervision is informative as to reflections of the patient's issues and the learning needs of the supervisee.

Supervision, and the manner in which the supervisor relates to and reflects on the presented material, whatever its form, models for the supervisee a process in which reflection, awareness, thinking about thinking, insight and learning can develop as an internal process. Supervision and supervisee development incorporates a process in which narrative competence and reflective function develops. Within supervision, it is the supervisor's ability to mirror and encourage reflective function within the supervisee about the patient that enables the internal development of these capacities. If supervision remains an environment that encourages exploration and curiosity in relation to the patient's narrative and conscious and unconscious communication, understanding and meaning will be created in relation to the patient and their internal world.

CONCLUSION

The impact of attachment is important in relation to supervision in order to consider, and be aware of, the learning issues of the supervisee as well as to understand the interactive dynamics that the supervisee brings to supervision and which may colour the supervisory relationship. Fonagy and Target reflect on this when they comment, 'Psychoanalytic training, supervision, and personal treatment remain crucial in enabling clinicians to use their emotional reactions to better understand their patient's subjective world, rather than be entrapped in the quicksand of rigid, unthinking patterns of relatedness' (Fonagy and Target 1998: 110).

When supervisees begin clinical work or start working with a new supervisor, attachment issues will affect the relationship dynamic. In supervision, where assessment in relation to training occurs, it is especially important that these dynamics are taken into consideration, particularly when there is a difficulty between supervisee and supervisor. However, I am not advocating using attachment theory as a diagnostic tool in relation to supervisee assessment but rather as a way of understanding the many dynamics inherent in the supervisory alliance, supervisee development and the development of clinical understanding.

It might also seem from this exploration that I am contradicting the points I raised in 'Internal states in the supervisory relationship' (Driver 2002), in which I indicate the importance of abstinence from the supervisee's personal world. In this present chapter, I am not proposing personal interpretations by the supervisor in relation to the supervisee's personal material but rather understanding in relation to the complex set of dynamics that interrelate within the dynamics and processes of supervision and which it is important to be aware of in relation to the supervisory alliance and the learning needs of the supervisee.

The attachment dynamics and internal working models of relationship will inevitably impact on the supervisory relationship, especially for supervisees new to the work, where anxiety is high and self-awareness low. Therapy, training and a secure and non-persecutory supervisory alliance will alleviate some of these factors and may, as Harris (2003) comments with regard to therapy, disconfirm attachment styles and motifs and hence engender a shift in inner objects. Supervision needs to hold a boundary between the professional and personal issues of the supervisee but be aware that the impact on the one will inevitably affect the other. In a healthy supervisory alliance, there will be containment, holding, non-persecutory appraisal, emotional processing and cognitive development. Providing the supervisory relationship can be maintained in a professional manner, this will have an implicit impact on the internal world of the supervisee.

Attachment theory provides a way of understanding not only the dynamics and manner in which a supervisee may relate and experience the supervisor and supervision but also the manner in which supervision and the supervisory alliance can impact on the supervisee and hence the clinical work. The aim of this chapter has been to begin to explore attachment theory, and the understanding that it brings to issues such as relationship patterns, internal working models, memory, narrative competence and the reflective function, in relation to supervision and the important components of the conscious and unconscious dynamics of the supervisory process.

REFERENCES

Ainsworth MDS, Blehar MC, Waters E et al. (1978) Patterns of Attachment: A Psychological Study of the Strange Situation. Hillsdale, NJ: Erlbaum.

Bowlby J (1981) Attachment and Loss: Volume 1. Attachment. Middlesex: Penguin Books.

Bowlby J (1981) Attachment and Loss: Volume 2. Separation. Middlesex: Penguin Books.

Bowlby J (1981) Attachment and Loss: Volume 3. Loss. Middlesex: Penguin Books.

Bretherton I (1991) 'Pouring new wine into old bottles: the social self as internal working model'. In Gunnar ER, Stroufe LA (eds), Self Processes and Development: Minnesota Symposia on Child Psychology 223: 1–41. Hillsdale, NJ: Erlbaum.

Bretherton I, Munholland KA (1999) 'Internal working models in attachment relationships: a construct revisited'. In Cassidy J, Shaver PR (eds), Handbook of Attachment: Theory, Research and Clinical Applications. New York: Guilford Press.

Casement P (1985) On Learning from the Patient. London and New York: Tavistock Publications.

Cortina M, Marrone M (2003) Attachment Theory and the Psychoanalytic Process. London and Philadelphia: Whurr Publishers.

Diamond D, Clarkin JF, Chase Stovall-McClough K et al. (2003) 'Patient–therapist attachment: impact on the therapeutic process and outcome'. In Cortina M, Marrone M (eds), Attachment Theory and the Psychoanalytic Process. London and Philadelphia: Whurr Publishers.

Diamond N, Marrone M (2003) Attachment and Intersubjectivity. London and Philadelphia: Whurr Publishers.

Driver C (2002) 'Internal states in the supervisory relationship'. In Driver C, Martin E (eds), Supervising Psychotherapy. London: Sage Publications.

Fonagy P (2001) Attachment Theory and Psychoanalysis. New York: Other Press.

Fonagy P, Target M (1998) Mentalization and the changing aims of child psychoanalysis. Psychoanalytic Dialogues 8(1): 87–114.

Greenson RR (1981) The Techniques and Practice of Psychoanalysis (second edition). London: Hogarth Press.

Harris T (2003) 'Implications of attachment theory for developing a therapeutic alliance and insight in psychoanalytic psychotherapy'. In Cortina M, Marrone M (eds), Attachment Theory and the Psychoanalytic Process. London and Philadelphia: Whurr Publishers.

Hawkins P, Shohet R (2002) Supervision in the Helping Professions (second edition). Buckingham and Philadelphia: Open University Press.

Holmes J (2002) John Bowlby and Attachment Theory. East Sussex and New York: Brunner-Routledge.

Knox J (1999) The relevance of attachment theory to a contemporary Jungian view of the internal world: internal working models, implicit memory and internal objects. Journal of Analytical Psychology 44(4): 511–530.

Knox J (2003) Archetype, Attachment, Analysis. East Sussex and New York: Brunner-Routledge.

Liotti G (1999) Understanding the dissociative process: the contribution of attachment theory. Psychoanalytic Inquiry 19(5): 757–783.

Main M (1991) 'Metacognitive knowledge, metacognitive monitoring, and singular (coherent) vs. multiple (incoherent) model of attachment. Findings and directions for future research'. In Parkes CM, Stevenson-Hinde J, Marris P (eds), Attachment Across the Life Cycle. London: Tavistock/Routledge.

Martin E (2002) 'Listening to the absent patient: therapeutic aspects of supervision'. In Driver C, Martin E (eds), Supervising Psychotherapy. London: Sage Publications.

Mattinson J (1981) The Deadly Equal Triangle. Northampton, MA and London: The Smith College School of Social Work and the Group of the Advancement of Psychotherapy in Social Work.

Perry C (2003) 'Into the labyrinth: a developing approach to supervision'. In Wiener J, Mizen R, Duckham J (eds), Supervising and Being Supervised. Hampshire and New York: Palgrave Macmillan.

Pistole CM, Watkins CE (1995) Attachment theory, counseling process, and supervision. Counselling Psychologist 23(3) July: 457–478.

Searles HF (1986) 'The informational value of the supervisor's emotional experiences'. In Searles HF, Collected Papers on Schizophrenia and Related Subjects. London: Maresfield Library.

Stimmel B (1995) Resistance to awareness of the supervisor's transference with special reference to the parallel process. International Journal of Psycho-Analysis 76(6): 609–618.

Stoltenberg CD, Delworth U (1987) Supervising Counselors and Therapists – A Developmental Approach. San Francisco and London: Jossey-Bass Publishers.

Szecsödy I (1997) '(How) is learning possible in supervision?' In Martindale B et al. (eds), Supervision and its Vicissitudes. London: Karnac Books.

Watkins EC, Jr. (1995) Pathological attachment styles in psychotherapy supervision. Psychotherapy 322(2) Summer: 333–340.

CHAPTER 6

THE EGO AND SUPEREGO IN SUPERVISION

ROSE STOCKWELL

INTRODUCTION

Ego psychology is one way of viewing the personality. It was, initially, a rather concrete way of thinking about the interpsychic processes within the mind, which involved the psychic agencies – the id, the ego and the superego – their development and interaction. As ideas about transference and countertransference, conscious and unconscious communication between analyst and patient and interpretation developed so too did ideas about the interplay between the ego and superego of one mind with those of another or others, that is intrapsychic communication. This chapter does not aim to be comprehensive but simply relates some ideas from ego psychology to supervision in the hope that it will stimulate further thinking. First, it orients the reader to the ego system. Next, it explores the interpsychic development of the ego and superego of trainee psychotherapists and supervisors within the supervisory process with a focus on the superego. Finally, it advances some intrapsychic possibilities where the dynamics between supervisors and supervisees could occlude the understanding of patients.

THE EGO SYSTEM

Freud's first topographic depiction of the mind is of a system comprising the unconscious, preconscious and conscious. His second, a structural view, describes three psychical agencies: the id, the ego and the superego. The id is 'the instinctual pole of the personality; its contents, as an expression of the instincts, are unconscious, a portion of them being hereditary and innate, a portion repressed and acquired. . . . it conflicts with the ego and the super-ego' (Laplanche and Pontalis 1985: 197). Associated with the unconscious are the primary processes of the mind, such as condensation, displacement and generalization. From a developmental point of view, the id is a given.

Secondary processes, such as thinking, judgement and reasoning, are associated with the preconscious-conscious system. These are adaptive processes, which enable an individual to respond to the contradictory demands of the external world, instinctual urges, the superego and the primary processes, and belong to the ego. The ego 'is that part of the mental apparatus where integration takes place' (Britton 2003: 91). Its functions, according to Hartmann (1950), include testing reality, delay of discharge, thinking and doing, recognition of danger and anticipation, and differentiating and coordinating. Added to these are the mechanisms of defence, which are described by Anna Freud as 'the ways and means by which the ego wards off unpleasure and anxiety, and exercises control over impulsive behaviour, affects, and instinctive urges' (Freud 1966: v). The ego emerges from the impact of external reality, instinctual drives and object relationships and is continually and dynamically modified by them. Its functions are further moulded and influenced by the nature of the conflicts and experiences each individual faces.

The superego is sometimes thought of as a subset of ego functions related to identification with and internalization of the conscious and unconscious aspects of the parents (imagos), family and wider social and cultural mores. Laplanche and Pontalis state, 'the super-ego's role in relation to the ego may be compared to that of a judge or a censor. Freud sees conscience, self-observation and the formation of ideals as the function of the super-ego' (Laplanche and Pontalis 1985: 435). The superego continually and unconsciously monitors the ego against its standards. Where there is positive appraisal, self-esteem increases with resultant feelings such as well-being and satisfaction. Where there is negative appraisal, self-esteem decreases with resultant feelings such as guilt, shame and worthlessness, and in Chapter 11 of this book Edward Martin looks particularly at the aspect of shame in supervision. The superego is a dynamic structure; to quote Freud, 'the super-ego, in the course of an individual's development, receives contributions from later successors and substitutes of his parents, such as teachers, and models in public life of admired social ideals' (Freud 1940: 378).

There are various views about superego formation. Some consider that the internalized parental prohibitions prior to the onset of the Oedipus complex are forerunners to the superego and that the superego proper is the product of the introjection of the Oedipal loved objects brought about as a consequence of the resolution of the Oedipus complex (Fenichel 1990: 102–105). Others draw on Melanie Klein's conception of an innate and pre-Oedipal, infantile or archaic superego emanating from the death instinct and being modified from birth. This pre-Oedipal superego is an aggregated organization, made up of 'a whole set of internal objects, each endowed with specific phantasy functions' (Hinshelwood 1991: 100), and which is modified through a perpetual cycle of projection and introjection creating good and bad objects, coloured by the id impulses. The good introjected objects contribute to helpful elements of the superego, and the bad introjected objects to harsh ones. In regression, these helpful and harsh elements may split and lead to idealization and/or denigration. Initially, Klein focused on the impact of the harsh superego, which she related to the early sadistic superego. Later, she described helpful internal objects, which corresponded to the infant's experiences of satisfaction, and which mitigate the harsh objects (Hinshelwood 1991: 94–111). Both views are drawn on in this chapter.

THE GAINING OF PROFESSIONAL IDENTITY AND THE EGO SYSTEM

Considering the gaining and modification of professional identity within, and as part of, the supervisory process in developmental terms is not original. The works of Casement, Hawkins and Shohet, and Enid Balint, for example, draw, in different ways, on developmental concepts.

Casement describes three phases in supervision. In phase one, supervisees have limited resources and supervisors provide a mental holding function and 'a form of control' (Casement 1985: 32). In phase two, supervisees have internalized their supervisors and increasingly think about their contribution as well as that of their patients to the therapeutic process. In phase three, there is what Casement calls an 'internal supervisor' who is in dialogue with the external supervisor in supervision sessions. Supervisees, in this phase, contribute their thoughts about the process of the therapy to supervision.

Hawkins and Shohet integrate a number of approaches from the USA into a 'combined developmental model' (Hawkins and Shohet 1989: 49) in which four major stages of supervisee development are described. Level one is characterized by dependency on the supervisor, level two by a fluctuation between dependency and autonomy, level three by increased professional self-confidence with supervision becoming more collegial and at level four the supervisee might themselves be working as a supervisor.

Enid Balint (1993) observed general practitioners attending 'Balint' groups. The aim of these groups was for the doctors to give verbatim accounts of consultations with patients to the group and seminar leader. These accounts were discussed psychoanalytically so that the doctors might, through understanding their personal responses, better use their relationships with patients. The scrutiny of their work by the group and the seminar leader put the doctors in the position of revealing themselves emotionally to a peer group and an authority figure while, at the same time, maintaining their ego functions sufficiently to reflect upon and apply what emerged. Under this duress, some came to use themselves and their responses to their patients more productively while others did not. Balint examined the responses she saw and identified six phases of ego development, which she equated to those known in childhood and adolescence. Phase one concerns over-idealization. She says, 'the doctors' introjected seminar ideas are superego introjects, unassimilated and not really identified with' (Balint 1993: 191). Phase two is a phase of defence where the doctor feels threatened in their professional identity. Compliance and rebellion and false solutions occur. Phase three is one of temporary withdrawal, phase four of assimilation, phase five of swings from compliance to rebellion and phase six of self-awareness. Balint considers that these observations had a bearing on psychoanalytic training where, as she puts it, 'the candidates are compelled to function simultaneously in two utterly different worlds: (a) the primitive privacy of the analytic setting, and (b) in the public professional worlds of their practices' (Balint 1993: 197). She felt that, caught in this dichotomy, many trainees remained in phase two for a protracted period of time both before and after qualification.

Elements from these models will emerge as the ego development of trainee psychotherapists within supervision is explored.

PSYCHOTHERAPISTS

Anyone wishing to train in psychoanalytic and psychodynamic work is already an adult whose psychic structures of id, ego and superego are developed. Recognizing this, most training organizations assess the personality of potential trainees to ascertain their suitability to undertake training and work psychoanalytically. In terms of ego psychology, the personal assessment explores ego strengths, weaknesses and defences, the nature of the superego and of Oedipal resolution. Where an adequately robust yet flexible personality structure exists, which can sufficiently tolerate and respond to criticism and conflict, training can be considered. Despite these endowments, training induces regression; this is usually most manifest in supervision where supervisors, willingly or unwillingly, unconsciously and consciously, are participants.

Recognition of this regression raises the question: 'Can professional elements of the ego and superego develop before clinical work starts?' An affirmative answer is suggested by the structure of many trainings where there is provision, in various combinations, of theoretical input, clinical discussion, infant observation, personal therapy, role-plays and sitting in on group supervision.

The manifestation of regression in supervision occurs, in part, because of the inherent dynamics of the situation. Trainees are in a dependent and demanding situation and are under continuous personal and professional scrutiny. This invites dominance by the harsher aspects of their existing superegos, which are yet to receive the contributions of their supervisors. Additionally, they need to gain recognition and to comply with the demands of their training organization. This is partly attained through their relationships with their supervisors, which unconsciously pulls them towards Oedipal enactment; wishing to gain favoured relationships and win approval.

In addition to the anxieties caused by the critical activity of the superego, there are others caused by the unconscious phantasies about psychotherapy and becoming psychotherapists. The professional ego skills for coping with this internal bombardment and for interacting with, and thinking about, the patient and the material from the perspective of the unconscious, are limited and depend upon personal ego strengths and skills learnt in former professions. So, when starting with their first patient, trainees are usually more reliant upon emotions and instincts to forge a therapeutic bond than on ego functions. A limited ego development may be evidenced by an incapacity to discriminate, an inability to know what to notice and what to ignore and by trainees being unable to assimilate and think about what is presented because they have no internal framework within which to link and process what happens. They may also lack the ability to recognize danger signals or to anticipate what may happen, and they may respond directly to the demands of the patient (Hartmann 1950). This experience of ego weakness or deficit can be overwhelming and leads trainees to ask anxiously, 'What should I do?' and, where critical superego anxieties dominate, 'Did I do it right?' They may lose confidence and fear they do not have the capabilities to be a therapist. At the very start, supervisors could be thought of as providing auxiliary ego and benign superego functions, helping supervisees think about and understand experiences with patients and giving aims, guidelines and models.

So how do therapists' egos and superegos develop from this position and how might supervisors contribute or impede development? Accepting Balint's view that professional ego development has similarities to child and adolescent ego development, one may turn to the processes of internalization and identification. Kennedy and Yorke's work on child development, applied to the supervisory process, suggests that the identification and the internalization needed for superego growth takes place only after 'certain steps in ego development' (Kennedy and Yorke 1982: 225) have occurred; specifically the capacity to generalize from a particular experience to new situations. For the supervisees, this would include generalizing from one session to others and from one patient to another. At this point, before new superego growth occurs and where regression is modest and the superego mild, supervisees direct their behaviour towards attracting approval and avoiding disapproval from their supervisors. But, where regression is severe an archaic, harsh superego emerges and more primitive responses occur. As Schafer aptly states, 'Before the final internalisation of superego contents we should not speak of a sense of guilt and conscience; there is only dread of discovery' (Schafer 1960:167). In other words, such supervisees fear that speaking openly will lead to the discovery of their having done wrong. The higher the fear of discovery, the more supervisees will struggle to remember what was said, how they responded or what they felt. Caught in a vicious circle, they can feel increasingly humiliated.

Internalizing new models involves a struggle in which the models have to be understood and accepted. The stimulus to start this struggle for children is the wish to be like their parents; for supervisees it is the wish to be like their supervisors. However, extrapolation from Kennedy and Yorke (1982) suggests three circumstances where this stimulus is diminished. One is when a supervisee does not respect their supervisor. A second is when a supervisor's narcissism causes their supervisee to feel disregarded as a separate individual. And a third is when there are conscious or unconscious discrepancies between the ideals of a supervisor and the ideals of the supervisee's training organization. In these instances, supervisees resist, consciously and/or unconsciously, the models and become compliant but not accepting of them. Their egos then develop defensively with a defiant undercurrent, and their superegos remain immature. This outcome corresponds to Balint's (1993) phase two.

However, when supervisors are respected and internalization goes smoothly, a healthy superego is established and, a modified quote from Schafer (1960) suggests, supervisees inherit wisdom and an internal source of self-esteem and confidence. (In this quote, the word 'supervisee' substitutes the word 'child' and the words 'supervisor' and 'supervisors' substitute the words 'parent' and 'parents'. Substituted words are shown in non-italics.)

> *From the adaptive point of view, the meaning seems to be this: the* supervisor *provides in the form of his superego, a pre-established structure for his* supervisee *to adopt so that the* supervisee *will not have to accomplish anew all the cultural achievements in the history of his group. A considerable psychic saving is involved for the* supervisee. *The* supervisee *takes over or internalizes this 'supervisor function'. He thereby becomes a* supervisor *to himself and acquires basic equipment for later becoming psychological* supervisor *of his* supervisees. *By introjecting the* supervisor's *superego, he also establishes a motivational basis for learning and perfecting a certain moral, protective, and comforting know-how. This know-how is part of growing up. In this process the* supervisee *is additionally helped to meet his ego ideal . . . and subsequently to feel worthy of love. And in being prepared for life in the community he is put in the position of being able to find, engage, and use alternative or modified real models and object relations such as he needs to complete his development.* (Schafer 1960: 183)

At this early stage, because of regression and the weakness of the professional superego, supervisees are vulnerable and particularly influenced by supervisors who inevitably pass on more than they are consciously aware. As supervisees' egos and superegos consolidate giving them a stronger and more mature professional identity, supervisors are less of a source of identification and internalization, and these particular unconscious dynamic processes in the relationship diminish.

As well as understanding how the development of the superego impacts on the supervisory process, there are situations where defences of the ego are prominent. For example, some trainees become enthralled by theoreticians and theory and persistently ask, 'Is this an example of what so-and-so (theoretician) calls such-and-such (theory)?' or report introducing to patients the latest theoretical idea they have come across such as, 'I told him that he was ambivalently attached to his mother.' In these situations, the emotional and instinctual are eclipsed, and the therapeutic alliance becomes an intellectual alliance. Contrariwise, some trainees, like some patients, are reluctant to develop their intellectual abilities and resist theoretical ideas for fear that this will block their emotions and instincts. Their ego develops defensively to protect their id. In supervision, they might say, 'I could feel he was near some strong emotions, and I intuitively knew it was vital for him to express this so I ----.' The ---- is something that is felt by the supervisor to be acting out, but it is defended vigorously by the trainee, often with a moral, superego, undercurrent. It will usually involve breaking a boundary.

As psychotherapists emerge from training and develop in their work, their egos and superegos become closer, and their superegos act in quieter and more benign ways as motivators, elements in reflection and boundary keepers. At this point, according to Hawkins and Shohet's model, they achieve a dynamic but stable equilibrium, gain increased professional self-confidence and may think about becoming supervisors.

SUPERVISORS

When psychotherapists move to become supervisors, their ego systems face further surges of development, which have similarities to those faced by adults becoming parents. They are again judged by colleagues or peers, either in reality through training or internally. This re-activates Oedipal issues and, where regressions are greatest, splitting of the superego into its ideal and hostile archaic elements occurs, sometimes with a projection of one or other of these elements into supervisees. Under these circumstances, supervisors are less able to use their ego functions, and specifically their capacity to know what belongs to whom is impaired. Thus, at the very time they wish to offer stability and wisdom, there is regression and fragmentation. These regressive responses limit free association and reduce their understanding of the unconscious meanings of what is happening. In effect, they are too anxious and are trying too hard to meet the demands of the superego and are not in a sufficient state of reverie for other unconscious processes to be accessible. Crawford in Chapter 4 explores free association in supervision and what happens when there are blocks or distortions. Supervision of new supervisors by experienced supervisors or consultation can moderate these situations.

Extrapolation from Schafer's (1960) paper 'The loving and beloved superego in Freud's structural theory' suggests that a supervisor's effectiveness increases as conflicts between ego achievement and superego demands are resolved and where they are, within moderation, satisfied with their functioning as psychotherapists. These factors make it more likely that they will gain the respect of their supervisees. By contrast, where supervisors' superegos are distant from their egos and where they are ambivalent about their functioning as psychotherapists, their pathology will tend to dominate, and the supervisee's development will be curtailed. In child development where the parents' pathology blocks children from resolving Oedipal issues, the results are severe superegos and a dependence upon the parents that is difficult to relinquish. In supervision, the corollary is that supervisees do not gain confidence in their own abilities and repeatedly seek reassurance about their functioning from external supervisors.

A healthy superego is flexible and adaptive. It is firm and giving, enabling supervisors to assert authority and to praise. Authority, when asserted, is given meaning by the ego and is congruent with the approach of the supervisor. A supervisor's capacity to be firm, perhaps overriding a supervisee's decision and insisting on different action, has the impact of helping supervisees reflect upon their impulses and balance, more accurately, internal demands with external ones. As supervisees gain confidence that their impulses are useful but do not need to be acted upon, they become freer to experience them, have less sense of guilt and are able to reflect upon their meanings. Supervisors with healthy superegos are genuinely pleased with their supervisees' development, which does not unduly threaten them, and any feelings that are aroused are processed. The expression of their pleasure in their supervisees' growth, verbally or non-verbally, adds to the confidence of the supervisees. To quote Schafer: 'Unconflicted gentleness is likely to go hand in hand with unconflicted firmness' (Schafer 1960: 185).

INTERFERENCE IN THE SUPERVISORY PROCESS BY THE SUPEREGO

The descriptions of supervisees' and supervisors' development indicate that the intrapsychic communication within the supervisory couple influences the supervisory process. Aspects of this communication can be thought of as transference, and, while weak transferences diminish as reasonable and realistic supervisory relationships develop, strong transferences distort supervisory relationships and the dynamics conspire against the transferences diminishing. These strong transferences therefore persist and interfere with the supervisory processes being used in the service of the patient. How can we advance our understanding and hence our responses to the transferences occurring within the supervisory couple? Symington and Caper have, independently, conceptualized unconscious and conscious ego system communication between therapist and patient in an interactional and intrapsychic way.

Symington writes:

> ... the patient and analyst become part of a system through which communication takes place. In his passive role where he does not assert his own view of the world the analyst allows himself to be swept into the personal-cultural contents of the patient's superego and interprets within that framework. Analyst and patient are part of a system and are joined through the superego parts of their personalities. (Symington 1986: 263)

Caper writes:

> When we speak of the patient projecting his archaic superego into the analyst, we mean that he causes the analyst somehow in reality to become infected, so to speak, with his archaic superego. The analyst's susceptibility to infection is a function of the strength of his own archaic superego: the patient's projected superego merges with the analyst's, and their combined force pushes the analyst into a state of mind where he experiences the analysis from the point of view of an archaic superego: not as an impartial scientific exploration of the patient's unconscious . . . but something else – a moral, or rather immoral, enterprise. In this phase of the process, rather than the analyst replacing a part of the patient's archaic superego with his ego, the patient has replaced (or displaced) the analyst's ego with his own archaic superego. (Caper 1999: 37–38)

Both Symington and Caper suggest that during the therapeutic process analysts slowly extricate themselves from an inevitable fusion of their and their patients' superegos. If we accept that, especially early on, supervisory settings usually contain influential unconscious dynamics such as power, dependency and Oedipal conflicts that are similar to analytic ones, we can suggest that in such situations supervisors' and supervisees' archaic superegos will fuse. This enables us to apply Symington's and Caper's ideas to supervisory situations, especially those where supervisees' transferences are interfering with the supervisory process.

Caper's ideas develop from Strachey's classic paper 'The nature of the therapeutic action of psychoanalysis' (1969) in which the idea of the mutative interpretation is introduced. This is an interpretation that makes explicit, at the moment of expression, the fact that the emotion, behaviour, attitude or fantasy being exhibited in relation to the analyst is displaced by an archaic phantasy object. Caper says, 'Strachey suggested that the internal object that the patient projects into the analyst in the transference is usually his archaic superego. As a result of this projection, the patient expects to find in the analyst something like an external version of his archaic superego, which is, in its negative aspect, harsh and punitive and, in its positive aspect, warm and seductive. As a result of the mutative interpretation, however, he finds someone not harsh, punitive, warm or seductive, but reasonable and realistic instead' (Caper 1999: 32–33). So, in supervision, where there is regression, we might expect the internal object that supervisees project into their supervisors to be either the negative or the positive aspect of their archaic superegos.

Symington's ideas suggest that in their passive role supervisors facilitate the receiving of projections, the interaction of archaic superegos and the production of fused transferences. Such transferences cause them to experience first-hand, albeit in an amalgamated form, their supervisees' superegos, and as a result they are highly tuned to their supervisees without necessarily making a conscious effort to be so. For example, a supervisee's harsh superego leads to all their supervisor's interventions being received as criticism. The supervisor unconsciously responds to this and, for a time, makes gentle and non-confrontational interventions. This gives the supervisee a non-persecutory relationship with the supervisor and decreases the severity of their archaic superego so they no longer receive all the supervisor's interventions as criticisms. Thus the supervisee gains the capacity to discriminate between critical and non-critical interventions and, as this more realistic position is gained, the supervisor begins to make the necessary critical interventions.

The example above is of a weak transference where the archaic superego diminishes as the supervisory relationship deepens without explicit intervention by the supervisor. However, where transferences are intense, the fused archaic superego endures and interferes with supervision. Consider the following situation:

> A patient deals with the rise in anxiety by a regression that leads to a split of the superego and the projection of the good object into a psychotherapist who becomes idealized. Unfortunately, as a supervisee in supervision, the psychotherapist has an enduring and unresolved idealized transference to the supervisor. The supervisee's and the supervisor's archaic superegos are fused, and the supervisee's idealization unconsciously gratifies the supervisor's severe superego. As a result, the supervisor does not see the supervisee's idealization and does not identify the patient's idealization when it arises. While this situation remains undetected, the supervisee does not appreciate the idealization of the patient and this does not enable them to take back their projections, leaving them diminished. Additionally, the supervisee is unprepared were there to be a collapse of the idealization.

Caper's work implies that the supervisors can become aware of the existence of these types of gratifying and defensive transferences if they notice a persistent, moral tone in their interventions or if they notice that they repeatedly think of obvious interventions after sessions. These transferences may also be picked up when the supervisor presents the work to a colleague, but this may not happen if the supervisor feels the work is going well. This makes a strong case for the presentation of all cases, particularly those that are going well or too well as in the above example. In these situations, the superego is stifling the ego, and it will only be when the supervisor thinks outside of the illusory power of the supervisory relationship that the nature of the transference will be identified. The transference then needs to be addressed and understood directly between supervisor and supervisee before the supervisory work can truly focus on understanding the patient.

One way this can be achieved is by supervisors making the equivalent of mutative interpretations to their supervisees. Caper links the mental processing required to make such interpretations to Bion's alpha function. He says, 'one aspect of alpha functioning must be what the analyst does when he is gearing himself up to make a mutative interpretation: he disentangles himself from the combined force of his and his patient's archaic superego, forgetting the supposed "moral" implications of his interpretations and simply describing to the patient what he experiences about him as realistically as possible' (Caper 1999: 42). He also comments, 'its [the mutative interpretation's] content seems very often in retrospect to have been obvious – at times embarrassingly so' (Caper 1999: 33).

So supervisors need to scrutinize and process what is occurring in the supervisory relationship in order to speak simply to supervisees about it. However, there remains a further hurdle to be overcome. Caper's work suggests that when the transference has been recognized and the interpretations or interventions conceived supervisors will be reticent about speaking out. They will become filled with doubt and fear that their interventions will spoil or damage their 'good' relationships with their supervisees. Their egos have to struggle with anxiety and guilt induced by their archaic superegos and to risk upsetting these good relationships, which may be particularly powerful where there is idealization. And it can be more difficult again where supervisors assess supervisees. In such situations, especially where negative aspects of the superego are projected into supervisors, the critical element of assessing enhances the anxiety, guilt and fear that supervision will be experienced as punitive and that bad or persecuting relationships will be promoted. This exaggerated persecutory element intensifies supervisors' reluctance to do anything that will disturb illusory 'good' relationships.

What can break the unconscious' prevalence in this situation? Symington (1986) suggests that intense moments of personal understanding can break the hold of these illusions. Imagine that the illusion of an overly comfortable supervisory relationship has been created by the prohibitive elements of the superego being defended against. The supervisor accommodates the supervisee, for example accepting changes in session times without exploration, and avoids conflict and confrontation. Employing the model of the supervisor, the therapist's relationships with patients are also accommodating and the negative transference is ignored. Following Symington's ideas, the illusion will be shattered if and when the supervisor suddenly has a thought, an image or a feeling that gives them the clue to their part in the illusion. In the situation described, the supervisor might suddenly feel furious with the supervisee for changing a session time and in that flash of intense feeling see the illusion that has been created. The supervisor then makes use of these furious feelings in order to show the supervisee what has happened and how this has impacted on their relationship and on the supervisee's work with their patients. It seems that in this intense moment the ego is freed from its subjection to the superego and thinking and understanding occur.

In summary, where there are mild superegos and regressions, the supervisory process can naturally, unconsciously and positively resolve itself. However, where harsh superegos and regressions occur, collusive situations develop that are difficult for supervisors to become conscious of and which require courage to resolve. While there is no resolution, the dominating dynamic of the supervisory relationship limits the supervisory process and severely restricts the understanding of the therapeutic process between supervisees and their patients.

CONCLUSION

In supervision, supervisors and supervisees reasonably share the anxiety 'am I good enough?' The realistic aim of this anxiety is to provide patients with a therapeutic experience that is beneficial. One way psychotherapists try to contain their anxiety is through seeking supervision, but in some circumstances this anxiety may be promoted rather than contained. This chapter has described some of the processes that occur in supervision in terms of ego psychology and indicated where and how these might be developmental or defensive. It has also offered supervisors some theoretical ideas to apply. It has drawn supervisors' attention to their part in some of the difficulties that emerge within supervisory relationships, in particular to be mindful that there are particular fusions of the archaic superegos within the supervisory alliance that are difficult for supervisors to become conscious of, without outside help, with detrimental consequences for patients, supervisees and supervisors.

REFERENCES

Balint E (1993) 'Training as an impetus to ego development'. In Mitchell J, Parsons M (eds), Before I was I: Psychoanalysis and the Imagination. London: Free Association Books.

Britton R (2003) Sex, Death, and the Superego. London and New York: Karnac Books.

Caper R (1999) 'On the difficulty of making a mutative interpretation'. A Mind of One's Own. London and New York: Routledge.

Casement P (1985) On Learning from the Patient. London and New York: Tavistock Publications.

Fenichel O (1990) The Psychoanalytic Theory of Neurosis. London: Tavistock/Routledge.

Freud A (1966) The Ego and the Mechanisms of Defence. London: Hogarth Press.

Freud S (1916-17) Introductory Lectures on Psycho-Analysis. SE 15–16. London: Hogarth Press.

Freud S (1940) An Outline of Psychoanalysis. The Pelican Freud Library 15. Historical and Expository Works on Psychoanalysis. London: Penguin Group.

Hartmann H (1950) Comments on the psychoanalytic theory of the ego. Psychoanalytic Study of the Child V: 74–96.

Hawkins P, Shohet R (1989) 'Maps and models of supervision'. In Supervision in the Helping Professions. Buckingham and Philadelphia: Open University Press.

Hinshelwood R (1991) A Dictionary of Kleinian Thought. London: Free Association Books.

Kennedy H, Yorke C (1982) Steps from outer to inner conflict viewed as superego precursors. The Psychoanalytic Study of the Child 37: 221–228.

Laplanche J, Pontalis JB (1985) The Language of Psychoanalysis. London: Hogarth Press.

Schafer R (1960) The loving and beloved superego in Freud's structural theory. Psychoanalytic Study of the Child 15: 163–188.

Strachey J (1969) The nature of the therapeutic action of psychoanalysis. International Journal of Psycho-Analysis 50: 275–292.

Symington NN (1986) 'The analyst's act of freedom as agent of therapeutic change'. In Kohon G (ed.), The British School of Psycho-analysis: The Independent Tradition. London: Free Association Books.

CHAPTER 7

SUPERVISION AS AN ALCHEMICAL PROCESS

CLAIRE ALLPHIN

INTRODUCTION

The supervision of psychotherapy is a complex and mysterious process that has a large component of unconscious communication between supervisor, supervisee, patient and the organization in which the training takes place. It is an intense relationship. In training, supervisees are dependent on the supervisor for a good evaluation, supervisors are dependent on supervisees for their good reputations, the organization is dependent on the supervisor and supervisee for the quality of work with patients and, of primary importance, patients are dependent on all three for help with problems in their lives.

To gain some understanding of the unconscious processes occurring in the supervisory relationship, this chapter uses concepts contained in the images (see pp. 101-112 below) from a sixteenth-century alchemical text entitled the *Rosarium Philosophorum* that Jung uses to illustrate the analytic process, in a book called *Psychology of the Transference* (Jung 1946). Jung became interested in alchemy when he was searching for the origin of psychology. He developed the idea of the collective unconscious – that there are universal images and experiences all humans share – and considered the alchemical text of the *Rosarium Philosophorum* to be evidence of these universal ideas about human relationships.

Jung (1946) describes the analytic relationship as a dialectic in which both therapist and patient are affected and changed by the relationship. Transference and countertransference are a combined process, and, through the involvement of patient and therapist, intrapsychic changes occur. Patients see in their therapists parts of themselves and through the therapeutic process eventually recognize these projections as aspects of their own internal world. The process is one in which consciousness is developed via the connection between therapist and patient and the realization of the patient's unconscious aspects through inter-actions, dreams, active imagination, free association, explorations and interpretation. The transference is primary; the connection is based on feelings that develop between therapist and patient, including the patient's experience of the therapist in relation to inner personal and archetypal objects.

Transference and countertransference also occurs in the supervisory relation-ship just as they do in the therapeutic relationship, and changes occur in both supervisor and supervisee without conscious awareness. Because the relationship is not primarily a therapeutic one, these unexpected changes may be threatening to the supervisee, as is the intimacy of the therapeutic relationship to the patient.

Jung used the concepts of the *Rosarium* to illustrate intrapsychic processes within analysis or psychotherapy, but they are analogous to the intrapsychic processes that occur in the supervisory relationship. The *Rosarium*'s images illus-trate a way of obtaining distance from the primitive nature of the therapeutic experience as well as the supervisory experience, and so supervisor and super-visee are more able to *think* about the process. It seems that Jung thought about these images as a way of gaining distance from difficult emotional affects in order to think about what was occurring in the analytic or therapeutic relationship.

There are limits to the extent that internal developments can be made con-scious in the supervisory process because of the boundaries that necessarily need to be held in supervision, since it is not an analytic relationship, though it may be, and often is, therapeutic for the supervisee. Our task, as supervisors, is to help the supervisee become curious about their personality and its vicis-situdes in relation to the transference and countertransference reactions that occur with the patient, and, if the explorations of the supervisory relationship are linked to the therapist–patient relationship, they will keep the focus on the supervisory task. The *Rosarium*'s images provide a way of representing a process, and an understanding of this enables a greater awareness of the possible inter-personal and intrapsychic dynamics involved.

The *Rosarium*'s images symbolize stages in a developmental process, occur-ring through transference and countertransference, and can be used to illustrate the way in which supervisees grow internally from states of being self-protective and hidden to knowing and integrating aspects of themselves as a result of their relationships with supervisors. Initially, within the supervisory relationship, the supervisee remains 'clothed', as in Figure 2, and is protected from awareness, but during the supervisory process the supervisee discovers and learns about their capabilities as a clinician. Supervisors may also learn about new parts of themselves as well.

This is a dynamic process and one which the *Rosarium*'s images can be used to represent. The images are not sequential and are presented here to illustrate dynamics occurring, at various times, throughout the supervisory process between supervisor, supervisee and patient.

THEMES AND CONCEPTS IN THE *ROSARIUM*'S IMAGES

The *coniunctio* (connection) is an important alchemical symbol of psychological development for Jung, and the images illustrate both the positive and negative, showing death and loss as well as rebirth (Solomon 1991). The overall theme is representative of connections and separations occurring throughout an intimate relationship that affects the development of consciousness. 'In supervision as in therapy we work within a paradox, loving and hating, holding and letting go, differentiating and synthesizing, giving and receiving' (Knight 2003: 46).

The first image of The Fountain (Figure 1) illustrates the entire process, containing within it all the elements that can be developed in either a therapeutic or a supervisory relationship. The remaining images (Figures 2 to 10) may be seen to represent an internal experience that is set in motion by an intimate relationship, such as the supervisory one. After the first image, the remaining nine depict a process that moves from self-protection (the clothed pair, Figure 2), to openness (the naked pair, Figure 3), to immersion in unconsciousness (the pair in the bath, Figure 4), to the unity or fusion of the two shown by the sexual embrace (Figure 5). This is followed by the image of death (Figure 6) when the pair realize their separateness after they have given themselves to one another. The image of the body in the sarcophagus illustrates the giving up of projections and defences. The homunculus leaving the body (Figure 7) represents the psyche leaving the body to become purified of its projections and is symbolized in the next image by the falling dew (Figure 8). The return of the homunculus, labelled 'Return of the Soul' (Figure 9), implies that there will now be an integration of body and psyche (soul), and this appears in the tenth image (Figure 10), that of the hermaphrodite. The emergence of something new (the hermaphrodite) occurs as the result of the death of old attitudes and assumptions of the supervisee, and so there can be an integration of new aspects through the learning process. However, if the state of fusion remains (image of the sexual embrace, Figure 5), supervisees are unlikely to develop their own internal professional and personal capabilities and will remain stuck in identifications and projections. This can be a problem within either the therapeutic or supervisory process, as Edinger (1994) and Ekstein and Wallerstein (1958) describe.

SUPERVISION AND CONCEPTS IN THE *ROSARIUM PHILOSOPHORUM*'S IMAGES

Images from the *Rosarium Philosophorum* provide a framework from which to view and consider the transference–countertransference in the supervisory relationship and to elucidate and understand the influence that the supervisor, supervisee and patient have on each another. There are differences in the way an understanding of these influences is used in analytic and supervisory relationships. Though these influences are often reflective of the analytic process, the supervisory relationship needs to be viewed through a somewhat different lens, that is transference-countertransference needs to be related to differently in the supervisory relationship than in the therapeutic relationship.

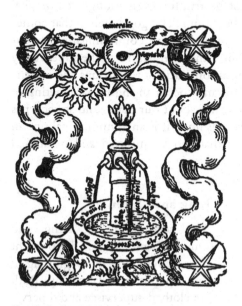

Figure 1 The Fountain

The Fountain

The image of The Fountain (Figure 1) represents all the elements (*prima materia*) of the relationship and the process. This first picture is considered by some to illustrate the entire process, containing within it all the elements that can be developed in a therapeutic relationship. The four stars, three spouts, two snakes and one fountain represent four to three to two to one and indicate the possibility of development from the differentiated four to wholeness, the one. This picture may be seen as representing the entire supervisory process, continuing throughout the work as a background, holding all the possibilities of what may occur in the development of the supervisory relationship.

In therapy it is the material from the patient and the patient–therapist interaction that forms the initial elements and these are usually more openly present at the beginning of therapy than they are in supervision as patients are likely to reveal more about themselves than supervisees. In the initial meeting between supervisee and supervisor, the experience contains many elements, but the two are differentiated from one another and each may wonder if the match will be a good one. How will this process work between them? Will the supervisee be able to learn from this particular supervisor? Will the supervisor be able to teach this particular supervisee? (Josephs 1990). The different ways in which supervisee and supervisor react to each other will be noted, consciously and unconsciously, by one another. Often the realizations that are seen and experienced in the initial hour will be forgotten until much later, perhaps when problems arise between the pair. This is a time of beginnings and each may want to please the other and/or to be an object of satisfaction to the other.

There is usually anxiety in the supervisee, especially if there have been problems with former supervisors (Brightman 1983). Supervisors may avoid being critical or judgemental at this stage in order to show themselves as good supervisors, the 'knowing ones', in their desire to be valued by the supervisee, just as the supervisee wants to be valued by the supervisor. Because there is the separation, as in the image, any discussion about the desire to please one another may not be fruitful, even though it may feel good to have such a discussion in the beginning. The good feeling that comes from such a discussion in an initial hour may ease communication, but it gives only an illusion of connection since the true nature of the supervisory work needs to include discomfort, separation, difficult revelations and internal shifts. There are also expectations that may occur in the initial meeting in relation to our prejudices. We need to think about our biases and stereotypes about people when we are in this relationship as it is an asymmetrical one in which we, as supervisors, hold power that can be misused and/or abused (Burke 1992).

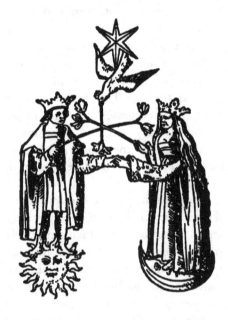

Figure 2 King and Queen

King and Queen

The second image, King and Queen (Figure 2), may be thought of as representing the beginning of the supervisory relationship. Both are clothed; supervisee and supervisor are not showing themselves to one another, and there is still uncertainty about whether this will be a good match. Their left hands are joined, which Jung says refers to an unconscious connection (Jung 1946: para. 410). There are many unconscious connections in the supervisory relationship. These include all three parties: patient, therapist and supervisor (Ekstein and Wallerstein 1958), the relationship between the supervisor and the patient and, often, the relationship between an administering organization and the supervisory pair. In the supervisory dyad itself, there are also projections, transferences and countertransferences. The supervisee may remind the supervisor of a previous supervisee, which may stir up associated feelings. Supervisors may remind supervisees of important authority figures in their backgrounds. These connections may not be conscious but can unconsciously affect the process and the dynamics. The clothed king and queen therefore represent the initial phase when much is hidden under the clothing (unconscious) that will come to the forefront for good or ill as the pair gets to know one another. I believe there are numerous new phases throughout the supervisory process, and, as each member of the dyad gets to know the other, there still remain parts that are as if clothed, or defended against revelation.

In this phase, the clothed king and queen may also represent an idealizing transference from supervisee to supervisor. The idealizing transference from supervisee to supervisor is natural and often necessary for the supervisee's development. The supervisee may need to feel a sense of power through being attached to a person who is admired and powerful (Allphin 1982). When this idealization runs a natural course, the supervisee eventually comes to a more realistic view of the supervisor and experiences their own sense of competence and power, accepting their own limitations as they accept their supervisor's limitations. However, when idealizing transferences are generated as a result of supervisors' needing to experience themselves as having all the knowledge in the supervisory pair in order to feel adequate, such supervisors remain 'fully clothed' and unconscious about their defences. This will then be reflected in the supervisee's relationship to the patient. The supervisee may express strong opinions and/or give advice to the patient in a process that reflects and parallels (Doehrman 1976) the way the supervisor has related to the supervisee. If, however, supervisors are able to examine their *own* inner experiences, they may be able to discuss these feelings with their supervisees, helping the supervisee to understand the effect on a patient of being with a therapist who needs to be idealized. This enables the supervisee to consider and dilute their idealization of the supervisor and think about their own need for idealization.

In the supervisory relationship, revelations from the supervisee may be disturbing to the supervisor. Sometimes complex personal information is revealed without any apparent consciousness of its meaning. When this occurs, the supervisor may become anxious about the supervisee's potential for development as a clinician. If there is material emerging from the patient that can be connected to a problem, it is not difficult to speak about the issue since it can be linked to the clinical work. However, if there is not a clear link, the supervisor may feel constrained not to speak about it.

For example, when a supervisee told her supervisor that she was estranged from her father, the supervisor was concerned about how this might affect the supervisee's relationships with her patients. When the supervisee was critical of a male patient, the supervisor was then able to ask whether there was any connection to the supervisee's life experience. This helped the supervisee examine her feelings about the patient and become more accepting when she realized she was projecting her experience with her father onto the patient.

In the example above, the supervisor's interpretation maintained the separation between supervisee and supervisor, but interpretations by the supervisor about the supervisee's relationship to the supervisor are inadvisable because there is no contract or container for them in the way there is in the therapeutic relationship.

For example, if a supervisee is angry with the supervisor, it is not appropriate for the supervisor to interpret this as relating to some figure in the supervisee's life other than the supervisor. At this point, distance is needed between supervisor and supervisee. The supervisor does not have permission to expose the supervisee to the supervisor's ideas about the meaning of the supervisee's reaction to the supervisor unless the supervisee has specifically asked for this.

In a similar way, if the supervisee brings up material about the supervisor, such as that the supervisor reminds them of their mother, this may be appropriate, but it is not usually appropriate for the supervisor to raise this. For the supervisor to question or interpret the supervisee's reactions in terms of their internal world or other relationships encroaches on the privacy of the supervisee and threatens the safety of the teaching/learning situation by making the nature of the supervisory relationship unclear. When such a confusion of boundaries occurs, the distance between the two, as symbolized in Figure 2, is lost and the question intrudes as to whether it is therapy or supervision. *Hearing* the supervisee's reactions, and being respectfully responsive, is an essential aspect of supervising.

Supervisees need their supervisors to be open to hearing about the supervisees' vulnerabilities, self-criticisms and concerns about their competence as they relate to the work, and supervisors need to be open to hearing criticisms about themselves from their supervisees. However, in the supervisory relationship, the supervisor would not be probing for revelations from the supervisee as the therapist might do with a patient. In the supervisory dyad, and in group supervision, much can be learnt about oneself in relation to reactions to the authority embodied by the supervisor (Cooper and Gustafson 1985). Supervisees' revelations about themselves need to be connected to work with their patients. It also helps supervisees relate to their patients' vulnerabilities when supervisors are accepting of their supervisees' vulnerabilities.

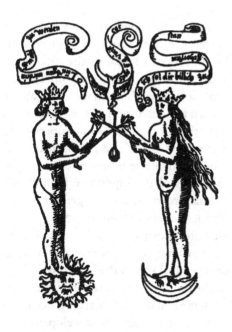

Figure 3 The Naked Truth

The Naked Truth

In the third image, The Naked Truth (Figure 3), the king and queen are represented as naked. In relation to the supervisory process and the ongoing development of the supervisory relationship, supervisor and supervisee become more open with one another. The supervisee may reveal concerns about the work, worries about competence and fears about making mistakes. The supervisor may experience feelings of not knowing enough to help the supervisee, or may become concerned about the competence of the supervisee, perhaps feeling judgemental about the supervisee's talents and level of self-awareness. It can be frustrating to a supervisor when a novice supervisee is overly self-critical and, as a result, becomes inhibited from using inner feelings and experiences to understand the patient in the therapeutic process. This is a time when the supervisory pair may become caught in negative feelings towards one another. When the supervisor becomes judgemental, the supervisee may become fearful and defensive and/or more inhibited. Recalling this image in relation to the 'naked exposure' of the supervisory process may help the supervisor modify negative judgements, thinking of them as related to discovering shadow aspects of each participant. The supervisor may be judgemental out of fear for the patient, and the supervisee may be defensive or inhibited out of fear of making mistakes and being negatively evaluated.

Self-disclosure is a complex issue, certainly in a therapeutic relationship, and also in a supervisory one (Burke 1992). I think of this image as representing self-disclosure in the supervisory process. Will the supervisor's self-disclosure be helpful to the supervisee? Since the supervisee is being trained to become a colleague, it seems appropriate for the supervisor to be more revealing than with a patient (Itzhaky and Sztern 1999). Sometimes self-disclosure is, however, in the service of the supervisor's comfort. When the supervisor is uncomfortable with the supervisee's idealization, self-disclosure may be a way to dilute the idealization. One of the complications is that diluting the idealization may be just what is needed in one case but may be premature in another where the supervisee needs more time to experience the supervisor as the 'all knowing' other (Allphin 1982).When there is a sense that the supervisee is caught in an idealizing transference or a negative transference to the supervisor, it may be appropriate for the supervisor, after self-reflection, to reveal to the supervisee the nature of the supervisor's inner experience for discussion (Allphin 1982).

Sometimes when I have felt tension in the relationship, I have asked about the supervisee's feelings about me.This has led to a discussion of the supervisee's fear of my judgement owing to their admiration of me.With some supervisees, this discussion, and my subsequent effort to show myself and my mistakes and vulnerabilities, has resulted in the person becoming more related and less inhibited; in other cases, the idealization continues and the supervisee is inhibited with me and with patients. In this latter situation, my acknowledgement of my vulnerabilities and mistakes intensifies the idealization (Allphin 1982).

Another difference between supervision and therapy has to do with vulnerability and safety. Supervisees need to be willing to feel vulnerable and to present problems about their work before they feel safe in the relationship. But I believe a supervisee begins to feel safe in the learning situation when they begin to learn. A problem needs to be presented, and, when learning occurs as a result of help from the supervisor, a sense of safety begins to develop. In parallel, a patient's sense of safety may begin to develop because anxiety is relieved when the therapist demonstrates an understanding about a problem, even if the problem is not alleviated.

With a supervisee, understanding is not enough for the development of trust in the supervisory relationship.This is another theme that can be illustrated by The Naked Truth.When the supervisee first presents a problem, there are usually feelings of vulnerability. The supervisor may feel challenged and exposed while attempting to relate to, and understand, the needs of the supervisee and the patient. The image can remind the supervisor of the vulnerability of this moment and the need to be aware of the possibility of anxiety in both supervisor and supervisee and the importance of acknowledging the experience of not knowing. This not only models the therapeutic process but also reminds each person in the supervisory pair of their humanness.

Immersion in the Bath

Immersion in the Bath (Figure 4) is the title of the next image. The king and queen are now in the unconscious and are relating without conscious awareness of the communication between them.This is a beginning of the connection, not yet conscious as in the next stage, the *coniunctio*.There may be confusion and disturbing feelings about communication within the supervisory dyad and between patient and supervisee. This may follow self-revelation and clarity about what is beneath the persona because there is now more trust in the relationship so unconscious material begins coming to the fore in both dyads. In the supervisory relationship, this may occur as a result of the experiences supervisees and their patients are having. Since much that is occurring is unconscious, the supervisee may not be able to articulate the problems with the patient, and so they are enacted in the supervisory relationship through a parallel process in the way the supervisee unconsciously asks for help or relates the patient's material (Ekstein and Wallerstein 1958). This unconscious process can occur in any

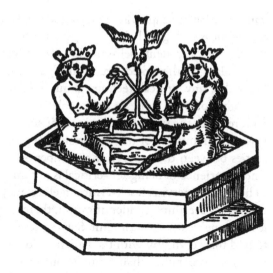

Figure 4 Immersion in the Bath

direction. Supervisees may treat their patients as their supervisors treat them or as the supervisees wish their supervisors would treat them. Or the supervisor may treat the supervisee the way the patient treats the supervisee. Or the supervisee may treat the supervisor the way the patient treats the supervisee (Doehrman 1976).

When there are tensions or problems in the supervisory relationship that cannot be understood, the supervisor and supervisee are immersed in their unconscious interconnection, very likely along with the patient. Awareness of this stage in the alchemical process may help the supervisor and/or supervisee to understand that unconscious material is in the forefront and that confusion and/or discomfort is a clue to a certain process that is going on between patient and therapist, therapist and supervisor and perhaps patient and supervisor. The discomfort or confusion may be thought of as information and unconscious communication from the patient and the therapeutic relationship that is being reflected and paralleled in the supervisory relationship (Allphin 1987).

Another aspect of the supervisory relationship illustrated by Immersion in the Bath occurs when supervisors have negative feelings towards their supervisees because they experience challenges to their self-esteem and value as clinicians and supervisors. When such feelings occur and supervisors are not conscious of them, they may respond to the supervisee in ways that are unhelpful or even harmful (Kleinberg 1999). An unconscious effort to maintain self-esteem in the face of challenges by a supervisee may take the form of becoming judgemental, critical, harsh, too directive and so on. The supervisor is trying to prove their worth as a supervisor and clinician and loses sight of the supervisee's needs and vulnerabilities. This can occur when the supervisee does not seem to be understanding what the supervisor is trying to teach, for example, especially when the supervisor is trying to help the supervisee be less self-critical and more understanding of the patient's self-criticism (Jacobs et al. 1995).

Thinking of the naked figures in Figure 3 helps the supervisory pair understand that any critical feelings about each other may be indicative of the possibility of open honesty being able to be expressed, and Immersion in the Bath reminds the supervisory pair of the unconscious nature of this experience. It is also a reminder of the importance of connections that are based on similarities between the supervisor and supervisee and the patient and supervisee. The experience of being self-critical is not uncommon in our work. Being able to hold the supervisee's self-critical feelings may involve staying immersed with the supervisee through identification, thereby experiencing the discomfort of feeling one's own self-criticism. Staying together in this way leads supervisees to find their own way with the patient through being joined in the agony with the supervisor rather than brought out of it through the supervisor's knowledge. When a supervisor imparts knowledge at a time when the supervisee is being self-critical, it can lead to further self-criticism for the supervisee, that is the supervisor has the (supposed) answer instead of the supervisee's finding the answer with the support of the supervisor. Awareness of the value of immersion with the supervisee may help the supervisor to not be threatened by identification with difficult feelings in the supervisee but rather to realize the potential for development and understanding when uncomfortable identifications are present.

The Coniunctio

Figure 5, The Coniunctio (the conjunction), illustrates the concept of joining. Here, there is more consciousness of being connected, and usually with good feeling. In the supervisory relationship, the two have come together and 'given themselves to one another' in a process in which both are affected, and often this is paralleled in the relationship between patient and supervisee.

In the supervisory relation-

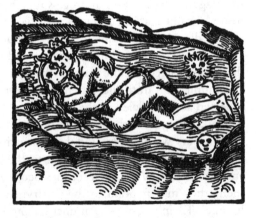

Figure 5 The Coniunctio

ship, the supervisee comes to the supervisor to gain knowledge of the analytic process and to understand about being with the patient. The uncertainty of the process often means supervisees need to join with their supervisors in order to develop the professional aspects of themselves that will allow them openness in the therapeutic work with the patient. It is a time when there is a feeling of closeness, sometimes an intense connection. Joining in the supervisory process is a vulnerable time in that supervisors may enjoy this so much they may not encourage the separation that needs to occur for the supervisee's development. The supervisee may also want to hold onto this feeling and so unconsciously will remain dependent and therefore hinder their own professional development.

This is also a time, as in the therapeutic relationship, when supervisor and supervisee are vulnerable to acting out the instinctual feelings that are aroused. Feelings of wanting to be friends or of being in love can occur in this stage as well as acting out in self-protection.

> For example, when an experienced supervisee came to me for supervision and described some profound changes that had occurred between her and her patient, I experienced feelings of awe and commented that the change was wonderful. The supervisee replied, 'You worked hard with me.' At this point I was aware that we felt very close and that we both had tears in our eyes. After the session had ended, I realized that I had finished ten minutes early and that my unconscious anxiety about feeling close to my supervisee had resulted in my acting out a premature ending. On reflection, I was aware that this enactment paralleled a process in which the supervisee's patient often made casual remarks at the end of their sessions that interrupted, and defended against, any intensity of feeling that was occurring between them. When reflecting with my supervisee, we were able to consider the power of the *coniunctio*. It is hard to sustain, a disappointment when it ends and difficult, at the time, to reflect on what it means. What was apparent, however, was that all three of us had an archetypal experience of unconscious communication.

The alchemical image of the *coniunctio* provides a way of understanding this particular dynamic of the supervisory and therapeutic processes and illuminates an unconscious tendency, within the supervisory and therapeutic relationships, reflecting dynamics that emanate from both patient and supervisee.

Death

The image of Death (Figure 6) is, I consider, a depiction of the experience of separating after having been joined in mutual understanding. There is a realization that an aspect of joining involves loss of parts of the self and disillusionment. The supervisee has taken in parts of the supervisor, and parts

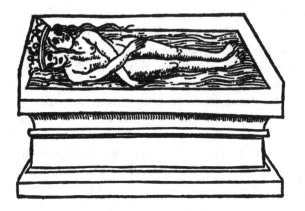

Figure 6 Death

of the supervisee have been turned over to the supervisor. This realization leads to the desire for separateness and this results in the loss of good feeling.

The two bodies, in the image, are one, with two heads, and they are in a sarcophagus. When a supervisee or supervisor has the experience of being different, of not understanding the other, of feeling critical of the other and so on, this can be experienced as hopelessness and/or ineffectualness on the part of either the supervisee or the supervisor. This is a time when the supervisor and/or the supervisee may have lost faith in the whole process, supervision or therapy. The relationship seems drained of vitality. This is a precarious time when supervisors may become overly critical of their supervisees and/or of themselves as supervisors. There is a sense of not being on the same track when discussing cases. The supervisor is in the position of having to trust the supervisee's work with the patient without understanding what is happening between the supervisee and their patient. This same process is very likely occurring between the supervisee and their patient. The image illustrates the necessity of recognizing one's separateness.

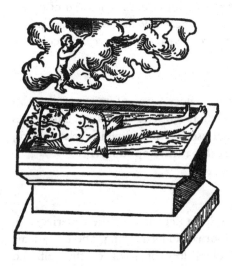

Figure 7 Ascent of the Soul

Ascent of the Soul

The soulless condition illustrated in Figure 7, Ascent of the Soul, may be experienced when there is no sense of a link between supervisor and supervisee. This image represents the soul leaving the body to become purified so that the body can then receive it in a clearer state, becoming conscious of unconscious processes without distortion. Thinking of this as the Ascent of the Soul points to the potential for change. Knowing this to be a stage in a process of development may help the supervisory pair to weather a difficult time, espe-cially when the supervisor feels concerned about the patient. It may help to realize that this state is one in which there is potential for change, that this death and soulless condition portends development for the supervisee and hopefully for the supervisor as well. In such a situation, the patient may be experienced as dissociated because of powerful feelings that are too painful to experience and, as a consequence, this is reflected in the experience between the supervisee and supervisor. The image points to the potential for change; consciousness of dissociation portends the possibility of a re-connection. When supervisor and supervisee realize the state they are in, it can be understood in terms of the patient's experience. When all hope is gone, there is the possibil-ity of the birth of something new.

> An example that illustrates this occurred when my supervisee talked about going fifteen minutes over the hour with a patient. I became flus-tered, could not think and felt alternately judgemental and stupid. I reflected on this and calmly asked my supervisee about her inner feel-ings with the patient. She commented that she had felt flustered and confused. It became apparent in our discussion that the extension of the hour was an attempt, by the supervisee, to get her bearings and make a link with the patient. The patient was someone who was dissociated from her experience and always talked in a matter-of-fact way about having been abused, which she did not connect to her feelings. I real-ized that in my initial response to the supervisee's presentation there had been no sense of linkage between my supervisee and me, just as there had not been between the patient and the supervisee. As the supervisee and I discussed this, it became clear that the patient needed to be dis-connected from her experience in order to talk about it.

Our exploration enabled the supervisee to understand what was being unconsciously communicated and enacted by the patient. The separating out of the supervisee's experience from the patient's enabled the supervisee to understand the patient's perspective, and as a result she was able to 'hold' the patient's feelings until the patient was ready to bring 'body and soul' together.

Purification

In the next image, Purification (Figure 8), the falling dew is purifying the body in preparation for the return of the soul. This might be taken to symbolize a time in the supervisory relationship that is more hopeful. Supervisor and super-visee may have begun to develop an appreciation of new strengths in the

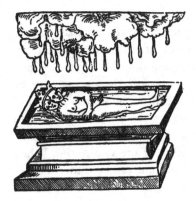

Figure 8 Purification

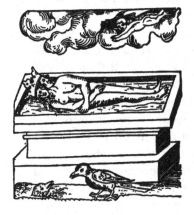

Figure 9 The Return of the Soul

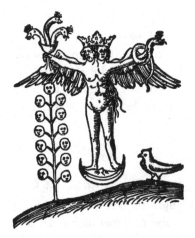

Figure 10 The New Birth

supervisee, and the supervisee may have a more realistic view of the supervisor. If the supervisor feels a loss of the good feeling that comes from being an admired supervisor, it may be offset by a sense that the supervisee has developed a sense of their own professional self as a result of the relationship with the supervisor and the supervisor's ability to teach and enable learning.

The Return of the Soul

The Return of the Soul (Figure 9) represents a return to vitality and more conscious realization. Within a relationship, such as supervision, there may be a sense of vitality between the supervisor and supervisee that is based on a new way of linking with each other. The supervisee may be better able to count on him- or herself, and the supervisor may admire the supervisee and feel pride in having been instrumental in this person's professional and, very likely, personal development.

The New Birth

The final image, The New Birth (Figure 10), shows a hermaphrodite; the two have become one. This represents the point at which, in supervision, supervisor and supervisee have taken in aspects of each other and each has become more whole. Supervisees have integrated what has been useful with their own talents, skills and sense of self. There is now a collegial relationship, a mutuality in which each respects the other's knowledge. They can each use the ideas of the other in their separate development as professionals. The figure represents the development of each member of the pair. Each has become a hermaphrodite, has taken in parts of the other to become more competent and developed as clinicians and supervisor. This entire process has a parallel in the therapeutic work with patients and reflects the themes of much of Jung's (1946) work and underlying philosophy, in relation to the therapeutic encounter, in that both participants are affected and changed by the relationship.

CONCLUSION

Use of transference–countertransference in the supervisory relationship is different from how transference–countertransference is used in the therapeutic relationship. Images from the *Rosarium Philosophorum* have been considered as illustrations of the supervisory process to assist in understanding developments in the supervisory relationship. When there are rocky times in the supervisory relationship, it is helpful to think of stages in the process; a process in which supervisor, supervisee, patient and often an organization are all influencing each other in their respective developments. Recalling the *Rosarium's* images aids in understanding feelings that arise in the experience as part of a developmental process to be viewed with curiosity about their meaning in the relationships between supervisor and supervisee and between patient and supervisee.

REFERENCES

Allphin C (1982) Teaching psychotherapy: the process of supervision and consultation. The Psychotherapy Institute Journal, Tenth Anniversary Commemorative: 17–22. Berkeley, CA.

Allphin C (1987) Perplexing or distressing episodes in supervision: how they can help in the teaching and learning of psychotherapy. Clinical Social Work 15(3): 236–245.

Brightman B (1983) Narcissistic issues in the training experience of psychotherapists. International Journal of Psychoanalytic Psychotherapy 10: 293–317.

Burke WF (1992). Countertransference disclosure and the asymmetry/mutuality dilemma. Psychoanalytic Dialogues 2: 241–271.

Cooper L, Gustafson J (1985) Supervision in a group: an application of group theory. The Clinical Supervisor 3(2): 7–25.

Doehrman MJG (1976). Parallel processes in supervision and psychotherapy. Bulletin of the Meninger Clinic 40(2-104): 1.

Edinger EF (1994) The Mystery of the *Coniunctio*: alchemical image of individuation. Lectures transcribed and edited by Joan Dexter Blackmer. Toronto: Inner City Books.

Ekstein R, Wallerstein RW (1958) The Teaching and Learning of Psychotherapy. New York: Basic Books.

Itzhaky H, Sztern L (1999) The takeover of parent-child dynamics in a supervisory relationship: identifying the role transformation. Clinical Social Work Journal 27(3): 247–258.

Jacobs D, David P, Meyer DJ (1995) The Supervisory Encounter. New Haven and London: Yale University Press.

Josephs L (1990) The concrete attitude and the supervision of beginning psychotherapists. Psychoanalysis and Psychotherapy 8(1): 11–22.

Jung CG (1946) The Psychology of the Transference. Collected Works 16. Princeton, NJ: Princeton University Press.

Kleinberg JL (1999) The supervisory alliance and the training of psychodynamic group psychotherapists. International Journal of Group Psychotherapy 49(2): 159–179.

Knight J (2003) 'Reflections on the therapist-supervisor relationship'. In Wiener J, Mizen J, Duckham, J (eds), Supervising and Being Supervised. New York: Palgrave Macmillan.

Solomon H (1991) Archetypal psychology and object relations theory: history and communalities. Journal of Analytical Psychology 36(3): 307–329.

CHAPTER 8

THROUGH THE LOOKING GLASS: CREATIVITY IN SUPERVISION

MARY THOMAS

> *The act of writing takes place at the moment when Alice passes through the mirror. At this one instant, the glass barrier between the doubles dissolves, and Alice is neither here nor there, neither art nor life, neither the one thing nor the other, though at the same time she is all of these at once. At that moment time itself stops, and also stretches out, and both writer and reader have all the time not in the world.* (Atwood 2002: 57)

INTRODUCTION

In this chapter, I will be considering some of Winnicott's theories on creativity and their usefulness in thinking about what enables or hinders creativity in supervision. What makes some experiences of supervision alive, stimulating and transformative, and others more deadly, with a quality of going-through-the-motions, or even persecutory experiences? I shall explore the relevance of applying Winnicott's concept of *transitional objects and experience* to the supervisory relationship, where the good-enough supervisor provides a facilitating space and the supervision feels like a responsive medium (Wright 2000) to the supervisee. I shall also look at less satisfying experiences of supervision, where creativity is inhibited or where the supervisor is experienced as persecuting and as the *impinging object*.

CREATIVITY AND PLAY

Winnicott's theory of transitional phenomena and transitional objects, based on his observation and understanding of mothers and their babies interacting with each other, laid the basis for a deeper psychoanalytic understanding of human development and creativity. He proposes a notion of 'primary creativity', a realm of 'illusion', which was the place of 'subjective' or 'transitional objects' (Winnicott 1951). He describes the essential feature of transitional objects and phenomena as the 'paradox' and the 'acceptance of paradox'. 'The baby creates the object, but the object was there waiting to be created and to become a cathected object', and 'we will never challenge the baby to elicit an answer to the question: did you create it or did you find it?' (Winnicott 1971a: 89). The baby at the breast, grappling with the me and not me-ness of the breast (mother), and coming up against the existence of an object that shows signs of not being under its omnipotent control, is operating in the realm of intermediate or transitional experience where the internal (fantasy) world of the infant is meeting the external real world. Winnicott believed it was important not to think of the internal and external worlds of the infant as in opposition to each other but to conceive of them as in the context of an intermediate space where these two experiences could be united and played with, or manipulated by, the infant, who, with the help of their mother, does not have to give up their magical illusion of omnipotence too soon, nor adapt in an overcompliant way to the demands of a too-intrusive reality (for example the mother's depression or other traumatic external realities).

This concept of transitional space, together with the experience of play in later childhood, offered a model not only of healthy development but also of human creativity. This challenged previous psychoanalytic perspectives on the defensive role of artistic creativity. Parsons (2000) explores Freud's contradictory ideas on creativity and his predominant view of the need to create art as a defence, which a person freer of neurotic conflict would not need. Parsons compares this with Segal (1952), who outlines a Kleinian view of artistic creativity that was operating more in the realm of object relations, seeing it as a reparative activity arising from the depressive position, when the infant attempts to repair the damage done, either in reality or fantasy, by its destructiveness. Both Freud and Klein took a more functional view of creativity, whereas Winnicott (1951, 1971a and 1971b) is interested in the nature of the creative process itself, and of its fundamental importance in early development. He believes that creativity first develops within the mother–infant interaction, before mother is experienced as separate and before destruction and reparation can have any meaning (Wright 2000).

Winnicott's view of the intermediate, or transitional, space is of a realm of experience in between mother and baby (or between artist and artwork), where the paradox of inside/outside, me/not me, fantasy/external reality could be tolerated and played with. His assertion that the baby should not be challenged as to whether the baby created the object (mother) or found her, echoes the descriptions of artists who talk of not merely having imposed their ideas on the material but of having responded to and expressed something that they found already there in the material they were working with. Michelangelo conceived of his sculpture of David as being imprisoned in the block of marble, and he was going to set him free. We may understand this as Michelangelo's projecting something of his own sense of being imprisoned into the block of marble, which he then liberates through the creative act of sculpting his David from it, but the important point is that it is in the *process* of interacting with his material that the work of art is created, which transcends conscious motives and creates something new and surprising, or an 'object transformed by subjectivity' (Wright 2000: 79).

Margaret Atwood addresses the transitional space occupied by artists and writers when she refers to the 'duplicity' of the writer. She sees the writer as occupying the real world and the pretend world at the same time, or rather a space in between, and uses the analogy of Alice-through-the-looking-glass to describe the transformative experience of occupying both internal and external realities, or life and art at the same time.

> *At the beginning of the story, Alice is on one side of the mirror – the 'life' side, if you like – and the anti-Alice, her reflection and reverse double, is on the other, or 'art' side. Like the Lady of Shalott, Alice is a mirror-gazer: the 'life' side is looking in, the 'art' side is looking out. But instead of breaking her mirror and thus discarding the 'art' side for the hard and bright 'life' side, where the 'art' side is doomed to die, Alice goes through the mirror, and then there is only one Alice, or only one we can follow. Instead of destroying her double, the ' real' Alice merges with the other Alice – the imagined Alice, the dream Alice, the Alice who exists nowhere. And when the 'life' side of Alice returns to the waking world, she brings the story of the mirror world back with her and starts telling it to the cat.*   (Atwood 2002: 56–57)

The looking-glass world has the character of transitional, or intermediate, space, where Alice can be herself and not herself at the same time, and can then return to her 'real' self transformed by the experience. It is this ability to submit oneself to an experience or a process, and to tolerate alongside each other the 'real' and the pretend, or 'unreal', aspects of experience that underpin creative endeavour, and the ability to symbolize. Parker, commenting on the psychoanalyst Marion Milner's work on creativity, observes the extent to which 'creativity depends on the ability to bear the ebb and flow between conscious and unconscious processes, and the capacity to sustain the conflict between individuation and involvement, emergence and embeddedness. She locates the tension between separation and union, internal and external reality, self and other at the heart of creativity' (Parker 1998: 761).

The ability to tolerate the tension between these conflicting and opposing elements, and the ebb and flow of conscious and unconscious processes, is also an important feature of psychoanalytic practice. A patient who can tolerate these tensions and has some ability to symbolize may, in the midst of a negative transference, rant and rail at their therapist in a session but then leave when the session ends and pay their bill. That is, they can tolerate the reality of the therapeutic frame, and also enter into the 'as if' quality of the transference, where a more disturbed patient, who is unable to symbolize, cannot and may experience the analytic therapeutic frame as persecuting, rather than as a benign transitional space. Target and Fonagy talk of psychoanalysis as a 'pretend' experience. 'Play is essential to it, just as it is essential to our model of the developing mind. Analyst and patient discuss fantasies, feelings and ideas they know at the same time to be false' (Target and Fonagy 1996: 460). Bollas (1992) also terms the constant toing and froing of work and play, and of reflecting and experiencing, that takes place between the two participants in a psychoanalysis as the 'play work' of psychoanalysis. Caper (1996) asserts that playing is an important means of exploring the relationship between internal and external reality and that an inability to play is a major handicap in people of all ages, since it prevents them from making contact with reality.

Winnicott emphasizes the importance of the ability to play in psychotherapeutic work, commenting that:

> *Psychotherapy takes place in the overlap of two areas of playing, that of the patient and that of the therapist. Psychotherapy has to do with two people playing together. The corollary of this is that where playing is not possible then the work done by the therapist is directed towards bringing the patient from a state of not being able to play into a state of being able to play.*   (Winnicott 1971b: 38).

He also asserts that:

> It is play that is the universal, *and that belongs to health: playing facilitates growth and therefore health; playing leads into group relationships; playing can be a form of communication in psychotherapy; and, lastly, psychoanalysis has been developed as a highly specialised form of playing in the service of communication with oneself and others.*   (Winnicott 1971b: 41)

If we look at the first of these two statements on play by Winnicott, and think of it in relation to the triangular nature of the supervision in psychotherapy, we could say that supervision is an activity where there is an overlap of *three* people playing, with the third present in fantasy in both the therapeutic and supervisory pairs. The triangular nature of supervision highlights and activates Oedipal conflicts, and difficulties in this area can seriously impede the capacity for play and creativity (Martin 2002; Lidmilla 1997; Mattinson 1981). It is important to consider the reasons for this because, in addition to the task of the therapist in enabling the patient to come to a state of mind where creative play can take place, the supervisor may have the task of enabling the supervisee to play with the therapeutic material or to engage more creatively in the supervisory relationship.

WHAT INHIBITS CREATIVITY AND PLAY IN SUPERVISION?

Or: on not being able to play

At the heart of Winnicott's (1951) concept of the transitional space is the good-enough mother who is sensitive and attuned to her baby's needs, and where there is a sense of a good 'fit' between baby's anticipation and mother's provision. In contrast to this, he describes another scenario where the mother is less in tune with her baby. She may be overanxious and underconfident and not able to hold her baby accurately in mind; a vicious cycle of maladaptation develops, and she is experienced as an *impinging* object. Sometimes a supervisory relationship can develop such a high degree of persecutory anxiety that little or no creative work can take place, and the supervisor may have the quality of an impinging object to the supervisee. As in a psychoanalytic impasse, a supervisory impasse or stalemate that inhibits creative play can be extremely difficult to unpick or shift and can involve many complex factors, including strong negative transferences and countertransferences between supervisee and supervisor, or between supervisee and the institution, when the supervision takes place in an institutional setting.

We could think of this kind of supervisory impasse as a *negative supervisory reaction*, much as we think of a therapeutic impasse as a *negative therapeutic reaction*, but it is extremely difficult to work with in the supervisory context, as the focus needs to remain predominantly on the therapeutic work with the patient and is not primarily concerned with resolving the negative transference of the supervisee. However, there is a school of thought – Martin (2002) and Szecsödy (1990) – which argues that, as the conflict has arisen in the supervisory relationship, this is where it needs to be taken up, as the conflict is likely to be evoked by unconscious elements in the supervisory material presented.

Anxious supervisors, perhaps not confident in inhabiting their own authority or believing that they are supposed to know, or be in the know, may, like an anxious mother, not provide a supervisory thinking space with a sufficient quality of transitional space. Or a supervisee, coming with his or her own particular history of internal and external objects and relationships, may not be able to make use of the transitional space provided.

Anxiety is an important factor in inhibiting play in supervision. Anxiety may be aroused in a supervisee or supervisor by primitive and unconscious aspects of the therapeutic work with the patient. The supervisor or supervisee may defend against the full impact of these primitive and potentially frightening aspects of the work by premature quasi-understanding, imposing familiar formulas rather than being open to new and unknown aspects of the patient's experience (Mollon 1997). Bion's (1967) advice to approach each analytic session with 'no memory and no desire' warns against a premature 'knowing', which closes down any thinking or exploration of the patient's internal world and their authentic experience. A further defence against the primitive anxieties stirred up in the analytic work is to defer or adapt too much to the supervisor, so that all the understanding and thinking is projected into the supervisor, and the supervisee adopts an unknowing or unthinking stance. A variant of this is when the supervisee evacuates excessive detail from the analytic session that may temporarily overwhelm the supervisor, and has the unconscious aim of getting rid of intolerable psychic pain, but has the effect of disabling or paralysing the thinking or playing abilities of both the supervisor and supervisee.

Other important factors that inhibit the ability to think and play creatively in supervision include excessive competitiveness, both with the supervisor and other supervisees in group supervision, and the fear of being seen not to know and the perceived potential for shame in this. Lidmilla (1997) distinguishes between a containing supervisory space where the desire to know is a mutual property of both supervisee and supervisor, and it is possible to have a playful understanding of knowing, and the more defensive and shame-inducing experience of supervision, where knowledge is felt to be the persecutory property of the supervisor. The desire to know about that from which one is excluded is inherently Oedipal. If the desire to know is denied, split off and projected as the need of the supervisor to know, the supervisor can then be experienced as intrusive and shaming. Lidmilla talks of a 'dynamic of shame' that is a feature of supervision owing to its triangular and Oedipal nature. He also states that 'the supervisory task always involves some *revelation* of a third hidden part, or an *inclusion* of the desire of the third' (Lidmilla 1997: 39) and that the third always brings together a pair. That is, the patient brings together the supervisee and supervisor, and the supervisor brings together the supervisee and patient. Winnicott's concept of the nursing triad can be used as a model of a supervisory triangle that is functioning well. The supervisor provides sufficient containment and back-up for the supervisee and patient dyad to interact in a mutually gratifying way, and the transitional space so vital for the patient's developmental needs is protected. If a defensiveness or collusion develops in the therapeutic dyad, the supervisor may be excluded and the supervisory gaze may be experienced as persecutory and intrusive, and thus be defended against. The supervisor in this situation can feel that the supervisee has created a smoke-screen around the therapeutic dyad, that they cannot understand what is going on in the consulting room and that the supervisor is the one trying to look through the bedroom door at the parental couple. The difficulty of this three-person, Oedipal dynamic in supervision was identified by Mattinson (1981) in her supervision of social workers. She was puzzled by the difficulty she observed in senior social workers' presenting their supervision work for supervision, when these same workers had no difficulty in presenting their casework in supervision. She concluded that the anxiety of the supervisors was due to the Oedipal nature of supervision, and that an important attribute of an effective supervisor is the ability to know about, tolerate and handle three-person relationships.

SUPERVISION IN THE TRAINING CONTEXT

Competition, anxieties about being assessed and being seen not to know, and the potential for being shamed and humiliated are all heightened in the training situation. The element of assessment powerfully affects the supervisory relationship and can feel like an unwanted intruder to both supervisee and supervisor. The production of an assessment report by the supervisor highlights the inequality between the supervisor and supervisee and represents something like an Oedipal third party (or 'father'), introducing an external, and sometimes unwanted, reality that might disrupt the comfortable supervisory dyad.

The heightened anxieties inherent in the training situation, compounded by the unconscious sadism that sometimes gets mobilized and enacted in training institutions, would lead one to conclude that this is where the least creative supervisory or therapeutic work is possible. Kernberg (1996) describes thirty methods that psychoanalytic training institutes use to destroy the creativity of their trainees. These methods or features include the systematic slowing down of the candidates' progression through the training, repetitive and unquestioning teaching of key papers by Freud and ignoring more contemporary psychoanalytic thinkers and literature, emphasizing hierarchical relationships within training institutes, discouraging any original thinking or enthusiasm in the trainees and cultivating a level of paranoid fear that will effectively keep trainees in their place. Kernberg describes the crucial function that supervisors perform in inhibiting the trainees' trust in their own work. This includes the supervisor saying as little as possible to keep the trainee in a state of uncertainty about their clinical work.

> *The candidate should feel that following his supervisor's advice without questioning and demonstrating to the supervisor that he has made the kind of interpretation that he understood the supervisor would have done will absolve him from severe mistakes in his work. This development will prevent the dangerous processes by which the candidate might otherwise integrate for himself a theory and personal frame of technique that evolves and changes creatively as he tests his views in the treatment situation while respecting the patient's autonomous development.* (Kernberg 1996: 1036)

Of course, what Kernberg is doing here in describing so clearly what inhibits creativity in training contexts is pointing to a different approach that would enable the 'dangerous processes' of creativity to develop more. However, despite the rather bleak picture Kernberg presents of the inhibition of creativity in the training setting, and despite the constraints resulting from the heightened anxiety, a lot of very creative work goes on in this setting, as the following example illustrates:

A supervision group in a training context, consisting of four supervisees and a supervisor, were in a despondent mood. The supervisees had recently received their end-of-year assessment reports. One member, Mark, had not received as good a report as he had expected. He was angry with the supervisor, and disappointed. It was Mark's turn to present, but he did not really feel like presenting. He wanted to withdraw. The atmosphere in the group was tense and sticky. Eventually, he presented some case material from his clinical work with a young female patient. He presented a last session before the long summer break, in which the patient was angry and disappointed with the therapist about his leaving her but was finding it difficult to speak about her feelings in the session. There seemed to be impasse all round, in the therapeutic session and in the supervisory group.

Eventually, as Mark presented the session, the patient started to speak through the soft toy she often carried with her, whom she called Foxy. Each time the patient spoke, she prefaced it with 'Foxy thinks' or 'Foxy feels', and, through the use of this transitional object, she was able to convey her feelings, and especially her negative feelings, about the impending break. The therapist entered into the spirit of the game and conveyed, again through Foxy, that he was able to tolerate the angry and disappointed feelings of the patient without being damaged by them. The imaginative use of the transitional object had enlivened the interaction between patient and therapist. It also had the effect of enlivening the atmosphere in the supervisory group where feelings of pain and narcissistic injury were now more out in the open and could be survived and learnt from, rather than disabling and paralysing the group's interactions.

In this example, the use of the transitional object by the patient had allowed her to express negative feelings towards her therapist, and to test out whether he could survive such attacks. The therapist's ability to enter into the playful exploration of negative feelings initiated by the patient, and to tolerate her angry feelings, helped to create a freer and more communicative atmosphere between himself and his patient. Also, in reporting the therapy session, the supervisee seemed to re-find his creativity, became more alive in the supervision and was freer of the persecutory anxiety stirred up by his assessment report.

FACILITATING PLAY AND CREATIVITY IN SUPERVISION

Given that anxiety is a major factor in the inhibition of creativity in the supervisory relationship, especially in training contexts, it follows that a significant task of the supervisor is to contain and alleviate anxiety. To paraphrase Winnicott (1971b), if one of the tasks of the supervisor is to bring the supervisee from a state of not being able to play to a state of being able to play, an atmosphere that is relatively safe and free from anxiety needs to be created in the supervisory relationship. This is akin to the kind of space for undirected thinking that Bion (1962) describes as being created by the mother's reverie, her capacity to be emotionally receptive and thoughtful for the infant. This state of mind and receptivity, which Bion calls the 'alpha function', enables her to take in and process the raw and potentially frightening aspects of the infant's experience, the 'beta elements', and then to present them back to the infant in a more digestible and meaningful form. Applied to the supervisory setting this process creates the potential space for thinking and playing with the material, both conscious and unconscious, presented from the patient by the supervisee.

Mollon (1989) describes the supervisor's task as being primarily to help build or create a 'space for thinking', a space for reflection, with a tolerance for not knowing and not understanding – a space for a certain degree of reverie in which peripheral thoughts, feelings and fantasies in relation to the patient can be brought into awareness and examined. Mollon's thinking space has similar characteristics to the intermediate, or transitional, space described by Winnicott as necessary both for the healthy development of the infant and for human creativity in all its forms. Mollon also states that the supervisor needs to provide a number of 'selfobject' functions, such as empathy, and quiet reflective consistency, in order to help create an environment that facilitates self-reflection and dream-like reverie.

NEGATION OR SUSPENSION OF DISBELIEF

Another important element of creating the optimum conditions for therapeutic and supervisory thinking and play is what Parsons (2000) describes as the negation of ordinary, or external, reality. Although negation can sometimes be an avoidance of reality, Parsons identifies the setting aside of ordinary reality as an essential element in all psychic work. Maintaining a psychoanalytic stance involves holding a particular kind of focus on the internal and psychic world and (temporarily) resisting the pull to engage with ordinary reality. That is, the analytic frame, the regular fifty-minute session, the frequency, the couch, the fee and the analytic stance of the analyst or psychotherapist all create an (extra-ordinary) setting where the internal, psychic reality of the patient can be explored. Within the safety of the analytic frame, ordinary conversation and social etiquette can be suspended in order to gain access to the internal world of the patient, and the paradoxical aspect of the play, or transitional, space, where things are real and not real, can be created. A suspension of disbelief is required to watch a play in the theatre, or to appreciate any other work of art, or to enter into a state of analytic play. Parsons describes the very serious aim of psychoanalytic play, differentiating between negation as a fixed state used defensively as a psychic refuge and negation as a temporary suspension or dis-engaging from ordinary reality, which 'makes it possible to work with the psychic representation instead of the real object, so as to come back to the real object in a new way' (Parsons 2000: 183). This dynamic is similar to Alice's experience of going through the looking glass and returning transformed by the experience, and with a new and different perspective.

In the context of supervision, the negation of ordinary reality is also neces-sary to set the scene for the focus on the psychic reality of the patient as conveyed consciously and unconsciously by the supervisee, and for a serious, and playful, exploration of the transferences and countertransferences within the supervisory triad with the aim of better understanding the patient.

Maintenance of the supervisory frame largely mirrors that of the psychoan-alytic frame, with the exception of the use of the couch and the frequency, and also that much supervision of individual work in training and organizational settings takes place in groups. Some supervisors adopt a more 'conversation with junior colleague' style, where more personal disclosure is encouraged, and may include describing case material from their own psychotherapy practice, ostensibly to illustrate a particular theme for the supervisee. One of the pitfalls of this approach is that the focus on the psychic world of the particular patient being presented by a particular supervisee can get lost, and this leads to more generalized hypotheses being arrived at in the supervision, with the danger that the specific meaning and dynamic of the patient's internal world may not be understood. Another pitfall is the potential for the hijacking of the supervision by the supervisor's unresolved conflicts or needs in relation to their own patients. The supervisor in this situation becomes an impinging object rather than providing a transitional space or looking-glass experience.

When the supervisor is working in an agency setting, there can be a pow-erful pull to succumb to the external realities that can threaten to crowd in and overwhelm the thinking, or playing, space of the supervision. The supervisor can feel caught between the demands of an agency to have a certain number of patients allocated to each therapist and the therapist or counsellor-in-training's need to achieve their required number of clinical hours with patients. The task of the supervisor is to tolerate the anxiety generated by these real, external, pressures while holding onto the reality and the meaning of the psychic work with the patients. In Kleinian terms, the supervisor needs to maintain the depressive position function in organizational settings where the paranoid-schizoid, part-object (that is hours, targets etc.) level of functioning is operating. In more simple terms, the supervisor needs to keep their head, or their analytic mind, when those around them are acting like headless chickens, overwhelmed by an anxiety which can be stirred up by the disturbance and need carried into an organization by the patient group. Given the power of the primitive anxieties evoked in such settings, keeping one's analytic mind can often be a difficult and lonely task.

THE IMPORTANCE OF THE FRAME

In order to create a space where play, creativity and learning can take place, the supervisor needs to establish a frame that is containing enough for the anxieties of the supervisees, stirred up by the psychic work with their patients. I am not talking here of the initial contract-making just in terms of the agreement of times, fees, setting etc. – important though these are – but more of the maintenance of an analytic supervisory stance and thinking that incorporates the negation of ordinary reality (as discussed above) and is concerned with providing a secure and consistent frame within which the psychic work with the patient can be focused on and explored. If we think of supervision as a potential playground in which the participants feel safe enough to play, the maintenance of the boundaries, or the frame, of the supervision is paramount.

Langs (1997) emphasizes the importance of the supervisor's management of the framework of supervision in enabling access to the more unconscious aspects of the therapist's work with the patient and the supervisee's experience of the supervision itself. Modifications of the frame, and emphasis on the cognitive and conscious elements of the supervision, hinder deeper explorations of the unconscious material.

Supervisees may present case material that offers a challenge to the frame-securing efforts of the supervisor, with the unconscious wish to see what the supervisor does with this challenge to the frame. This is similar to the patient who tests the boundaries of the psychotherapist in order to find out if they are in safe hands, and whether they will be able to feel contained. Sometimes, gross challenges to the frame are presented in supervision which inhibit creative therapeutic work in that all the energy goes into efforts to secure the frame.

FINDING THE OBJECT THAT IS WAITING TO BE CREATED

In a sense, one could describe all psychoanalytic supervision as directed towards the aim of finding the object that is waiting to be found or created. The supervisee presents the verbatim report, or memory, of the clinical session with a patient, and the supervisor, or supervisor and supervision group, listen and reflect on the material presented, and notice and comment on their associations, thoughts or feelings stirred up in response to the clinical material and the experience of the presentation. If all goes well and there is a good-enough working alliance between supervisee and supervisor, or supervision group, all participants might feel that they have been engaged in a process that has created a new 'object', which might be a new understanding of the patient and his or her internal world and quality of object relating.

The supervisee comes with the written report of the clinical session, which might be thought of as the script of the play about to unfold. There the analogy ends, unless one conceives of a play with a high degree of improvisation and audience participation which is being continuously transformed by the audience so that every performance is unique and different. The report of the clinical session is the raw material that is subjectively transformed within the context of the supervisory relationship into a more processed, or 'cooked', and more easily understandable and digestible form. This is an important function for the therapist working with patients with borderline psychopathologies, where there is a high level of unconscious, primitive and destructive projections operating, which may make it difficult for the therapist to maintain their capacity for thinking in the clinical situation. I do not want to carry the cooking analogy too far, though, as there may be a danger of overcooking, of premature knowing or theorizing which forecloses new and surprising insights or ideas. To maintain the creative quality of the transitional space, the supervisor and supervisee need to inhabit an attitude of being open to the experience in the supervision, and to the thoughts and feelings stirred up by the clinical material, and be able to play with the new material, or 'objects', that come out of the experience. Out of the creative intercourse comes the third – the new idea, insight or understanding.

Ideally, the receptive and creative atmosphere in the supervisory relationship models and feeds into the supervisee's clinical work and contributes to the potential for discovering new understandings, or 'objects', waiting to be found in the therapeutic work. This was clearly evident in the following example:

> A supervisee presented a session with a patient. The patient was threatening to leave her partner, and the supervisee became concerned and preoccupied with how this would affect the patient's baby daughter. The supervisee spoke in very conscious and cognitive terms, somewhat out

of character, and as the presentation went on the supervisor felt more and more uncomfortable and anxious. The supervisee then reported having a sneezing fit, which seemed to come from nowhere, and which had happened before with this patient. After reporting this, the supervisee returned to his very conscious presentation, with seemingly no curiosity about the sneezing fit, or its possible meanings. The supervisor intervened at this point, feeling that there was a link between her sense of mounting anxiety during the presentation and the sneezing fit, as if the primitive and preverbal anxieties of the patient were breaking through the conscious defences in the sneezing fit and trying to make themselves heard; although the supervisee, at that point, was finding it difficult to hear.

After discussion of the patient's unconscious communications, especially as manifested in the sneezing fit, and the supervisor's sense of anxiety during the overly conscious presentation, a new understanding of the supervisee's preoccupation with the patient's actual baby was reached. It stood in for, but also protected the supervisee against, the full force of the uncontained baby-self of the patient in the room. The symbolic baby waiting to be found was found through the experience of the supervision, and the anxieties communicated by the uncontained baby could be more tolerated and heard in the thinking space, or transitional space, of the supervision.

PLAYING WITH WORDS

Thinking about the clinical material presented in supervision imaginatively, through word play and use of metaphor, can free up creative blocks and impasses in the therapeutic or supervisory setting. Ogden comments that without metaphor we are stuck in a world of surfaces with meanings that cannot be reflected on, and that 'the analytic use of reverie is the process by which unconscious experience is made into verbally symbolic metaphors that re-present unconscious aspects of ourselves to ourselves' (Ogden 1997: 727).

A metaphor is a means of saying one thing in terms of another and could be thought of as a kind of transitional object that enables meaning to be communicated. In contrast to clichés, where experience is drained of meaning by being squeezed into formulaic and predictable assumptions, metaphors have the potential to open up possibilities about the meaning of experience.

For example, a patient who struggled to convey her despairing and lethargic state of mind eventually came up with the metaphor of feeling like a sack of potatoes. The therapist and patient were able to play with this metaphor, exploring the particular qualities of a sack of potatoes and how these related to the patient's feelings about herself, and this led onto more thoughts and understanding of the patient's internal world.

In the context of supervision, playing with the words produced by the patient, especially where the patient is concrete (non-metaphorical) in their thinking, can help to deepen understanding of the patient's unconscious communications and enable the supervisee and supervisor to return, like Alice, with a new understanding.

CONCLUSION

In this chapter, I have outlined some thoughts about what factors contribute to enabling or hindering creativity in supervision. Creativity cannot be manufactured, and any lack of creativity in supervision, like the 'creative blocks' that artists and writers experience, may be due to many complex internal and unconscious factors brought to the supervisory relationship by the supervisor, supervisee and patient. My focus has been on the nature of the supervisory relationship and the importance of the provision of a quality of transitional space, within a secure frame, that enables the play-work of supervision to take place.

To enter into the state of creative play, there needs to be an emotional and intellectual openness to its paradoxical nature, a toleration of moving between the real and the pretend, and of the ebb and flow of conscious and unconscious processes. Like Alice, who was transformed by her journey through the looking glass, and the strange and surprising experiences she had there, the supervisory pair, or group, need to engage in a suspension of disbelief or negation of ordinary reality in order to be open to the unconscious communication from the patient and to find the object waiting to be found or created.

REFERENCES

Atwood M (2002) Negotiating with the Dead: A Writer on Writing. Cambridge: Cambridge University Press. © O.W. Toad Ltd. 2002.

Bion WR (1962) Learning from Experience. London: Heinemann.

Bion WR (1967) Second Thoughts. London: Heinemann.

Bollas C (1992) Being a Character: Psychoanalysis and Self Experience. London: Routledge.

Caper R (1996) Play, experimentation and creativity. International Journal of Psycho-Analysis 77(5): 859–869.

Kernberg O (1996) Thirty methods to destroy the creativity of psychoanalytic candidates. International Journal of Psycho-Analysis 77(5): 1031–1040.

Langs R (1997) 'The framework of supervision in psychoanalytic psychotherapy'. In
    Martindale B et al. (eds), Supervision and its Vicissitudes. London: Karnac Books.
Lidmilla A (1997) 'Shame, knowledge and modes of enquiry in supervision'. In Shipton G
    (ed.), Supervision of Psychotherapy and Counselling: Making a Place to Think.
    Buckingham: Open University Press.
Martin E (2002) 'Listening to the absent patient: therapeutic aspects of supervision'. In Driver
    C, Martin E (eds), Supervising Psychotherapy: Psychoanalytic and Psychodynamic
    Perspectives. London: Sage Publications.
Mattinson J (1975) The Reflection Process in Casework Supervision. London: Tavistock
    Institute of Marital Studies.
Mattinson J (1981) The Deadly Equal Triangle. Northampton, MA, and London: The Smith
    College School of Social Work and the Group of the Advancement of Psychotherapy in
    Social Work.
Mollon P (1989) Anxiety, supervision and a space for thinking: some narcissistic perils for
    clinical psychologists in learning psychotherapy. British Journal of Medical Psychology 62:
    113–22.
Mollon P (1997) 'Supervision as a space for thinking'. In Shipton G (ed.), Supervision of
    Psychotherapy and Counselling: Making a Place to Think. Buckingham: Open University
    Press.
Ogden T (1997) Reverie and metaphor. International Journal of Psycho-Analysis 78(4):
    719–732.
Parker R (1998) Killing the angel in the house: creativity, femininity and aggression.
    International Journal of Psycho-Analysis 79(4): 757–774.
Parsons M (2000) The Dove that Returns, The Dove that Vanishes: Paradox and Creativity in
    Psychoanalysis. London: Routledge.
Segal H (1952) 'A psycho-analytical approach to aesthetics'. In The Work of Hanna Segal
    (1980) 185–206. New York: Jason Aronson.
Szecsödy I (1990) Supervision: a didactic or mutative situation. Psychoanalytic Psychotherapy
    4(3): 245–262.
Target M, Fonagy P (1996) Playing with Reality II. International Journal of Psycho-Analysis
    77(3): 459–479.
Winnicott DW (1951) 'Transitional objects and transitional phenomena'. In Through
    Paediatrics to Psychoanalysis. London: Hogarth Press (reprinted London: Karnac Books,
    1992).
Winnicott DW (1971a) 'The use of an object'. In Playing and Reality. London: Tavistock
    (reprinted London: Routledge, 1991)
Winnicott DW (1971b) 'Playing: a theoretical statement'. In Playing and Reality. London:
    Tavistock (reprinted London: Routledge, 1996).
Wright K (2000) 'To make experience sing'. In Caldwell L (ed.) Art, Creativity, Living.
    London: Karnac Books.

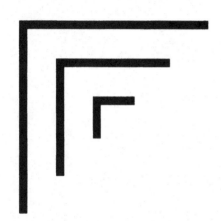

SECTION III

INTERDISCIPLINARY
DIALOGUES

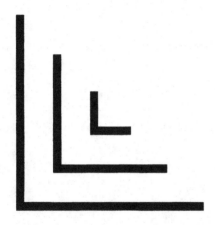

CHAPTER 9
SUPERVISION AND TRAINING: TWO DIFFERENT FOCI

SANDRA THOMAS

INTRODUCTION

The art of psychotherapy evolves out of a complex system. It requires creative and imaginative thinking, knowledge of a theoretical modality, intelligence, the ability to formulate and communicate ideas, intuitive understanding of the patient's internal world and empathy. The art of the psychotherapist rests upon this system. The question of whether and how this art can be taught, and how much the trainee and professional practitioner brings of themselves to the work, is a key question in training and, indeed, for the selection process for psychotherapy training. In other words, is the art of the practitioner innate or developed through the rigours of training, learning and supervision?

The demands of training require that the trainee internalize and integrate theory in relation to practice through the dynamics of lectures and theoretical input, personal training therapy and the supervision of clinical work undertaken as part of the training programme. The trainee, therefore, stands at the centre of a complex dynamic of interacting forces of both a conscious and unconscious nature of which, through processes of integration and insight, the trainee has to make sense in order to assimilate theory and practice. Supervision is but one of these interacting forces, and the emphasis upon its experiential and dynamic nature is widely acknowledged. Supervision has variously been defined as 'a chance to stand back and reflect' (Hawkins and Shohet 2002: 3), a relationship based on the need to understand another, the patient (Driver 2002), and 'a reflection process which may offer clues to obscure difficulties besetting the patient–therapist relationship' (Searles 1955: 159). For the supervisee within training, it is this dual process of assimilation and insight, and its conscious and unconscious affect within supervision, that is key to the trainee's clinical learning and development.

This chapter will examine some of the requirements and dynamics of training, how inner and outer reality can become caught within the supervisory relationship and how supervision, the supervisor and supervisee have to hold the tension between the two different, but interrelated, foci of the needs of the patient and the needs of the training and, within these, the personal needs of the supervisee. The chapter will also reflect the nature of clinical responsibility and how this can create a tension between the different elements of the training and consider how the relationship between supervisors, seminar leaders, course organizers and training committees can be best enhanced.

REFLECTIONS UPON THE HISTORY OF TRAINING

Forms and modes of psychotherapeutic training have a long history that predates the early twentieth century. The struggle to establish a recognized form of training was not without its political antagonists and seemed to represent those early primitive processes familiar to the analyst and implicit in psychoanalytic treatment. The structure of psychoanalytic training was first organized at the Berlin Institute between 1922 and 1924. Called the Eitington model, it composed a training analysis, a theoretical component and supervision of selected training patients. In its conception, this reflected the Oedipal constellations of Freudian theory and was in direct contrast to object-relations constellations of the Hungarian model where therapy and supervision were conducted by the same analyst. The analyses of the Eitington model were called didactic to differentiate them from ordinary therapeutic analysis, and the analysis of trainees was the province only of a small elite group called training analysts. It was believed that this essential part of the training process became internalized into the trainee's unconscious, influencing both style and practice. Completion of the tripartite requirements of training did not automatically bestow graduation or entitlement upon the trainees. It was envisaged that the newly qualified practitioner, no longer restricted by the requirements of training, its scrutiny and examination, and in a transitional phase of maturation, would cling to an analytic discipline as a defence against separation anxiety. However, this same analytic discipline created a paradox whereby unconscious injuries stimulated by, and inherent within, a training programme, and felt by the inexperienced trainee, remained unresolved and embedded within the internal world of the trainee during the training and after it.

Whether in the historical past or the present day, 'training institutes often function on the basis of unresolved transference relations and, whilst the therapist is supposed to help the patient resolve the transference, the practitioner's transference is often being manipulated by the demands of the training' (Roustang 1982: 20). Early criticisms of this approach concerned the dangers of a too rigorous psychoanalytic orthodoxy. Balint argues that 'the general aim of any initiation rite forces the candidate to identify himself with his initiator, to introject the behaviour as well as the working of the training system, which has several features leading to a weakening of ego functions, and to the formation and strengthening of a special kind of superego' (Balint 1948: 167). The thrust of Balint's argument is that, where superego dynamics operate to condition the practitioner's sense of their integrity as a therapist, the important focus of any supervision must be on encouraging the practitioner to listen to their own countertransference reaction and to interpret the transference of the patient within the context of the material presented. From this it would seem that a requirement of supervision was that the supervisor consider and understand the impact of the demands and transference issues emanating from the training alongside those emanating from the patient. Thus, by the second half of the last century, there had been a significant shift from the simplistic training analysis towards a complex interacting dynamic that involved a consideration of many factors which are still pertinent in contemporary training programmes.

THE AIMS AND FOCI OF TRAINING

Within psychodynamic work, the issue of how to understand the mental life of the patient draws heavily upon the use of symbolism and metaphor and the finding of meaning with, and for, the patient. Freud wrote that psychoanalysts – and here are included psychoanalytic psychotherapists and psychodynamic counsellors – are marked by a particularly strict belief in the determination of mental life. 'For them there is nothing trivial, nothing arbitrary or haphazard . . . the discipline of psychoanalytic work is in the seeking to bring to conscious recognition the things in mental life which are repressed; and everyone who forms a judgement on it is himself a human being, who possesses similar repressions' (Freud 1909: 67).

The commonalities between trainee and experienced practitioner highlight certain aspects of methodology, such as the theoretical and technical concepts that condition the form and mode of psychoanalytic work, the capacity to use symbolism and metaphor and the implications of creating a permanence of setting. The processes of training, therefore, require that a trainee become more conscious of internal processes and develop from concrete modes of operation and thinking to symbolic modes of reflection. The capacity to move from thing presentation to word presentation and from concrete operational thought to symbolic modes of functioning is fundamental to the development of the professional practitioner. And yet this same capacity to shift from one operational method to another will in itself create intense anxiety in the trainee.

In the process of the learning experience is an accompanying disturbance of the sense of self. In a 'Piagetian sense, learning involves the process of both assimilation and accommodation of new experience; and it is the latter which creates the anxieties as the learner questions existing schemata and alters style to include new knowledge and experience' (Thomas 1997: 72). In addition, training also requires the curiosity of the trainees and their ability to develop the capacity to experience the processes of splitting, projective identification and unconscious communication from the patient. The understanding and interpretation of unconscious symbolism is one of the main tools of the psychotherapist, who is often faced with the task of understanding and recognizing the meaning not only of a particular symbol but also of the whole process of symbol formation (Segal 1986). In a developmental sense, if symbolization does not occur, the whole development of the ego is arrested, and this affects not only the 'whole foundation of phantasy and sublimation, but more than that, the basis of the subject's relations to the outside world and to reality in general' (Klein 1930: 97). Training, therefore, requires the trainee to develop symbolic activity and to be able to move from paranoid-schizoid projective states to being able to hold and contain within the depressive position.

Supervision is concerned with the exploration of the intersubjective and the intrasubjective experience of the encounter as it unfolds in the supervisory dialogue between the trainee and the supervisor. The supervisory triangulation of the therapeutic dyad, enables a diminishing in intensity of the primitive processes that can get caught up in a dyad and enables a thinking space to be established in which the trainee may come to recognize the symbolic meaning of the encounter with the patient. In supervision, constant vigilance is given to the primitive processes and the unpacking of their symbolic meaning, with particular attention favouring the close-up analysis of the transference and countertransference.

The supervisor listens to all the prime ingredients of the trainee's material and associations as presented, considers their responses to the interventions and translates the material, looking for the pertinent signs that give symbolic meaning in relation to the patient and the patient–therapist relationship. The supervisor then puts these reflections to good use, highlighting any enactments within the supervisory encounter which may parallel the processes that are operant within the therapeutic setting. For instance, 'a supervisor's capacity to think about how the therapist can be pulled into an enactment and what this may be defending against is vital since it triangulates the interaction' (Lloyd-Owen 2003: 293).

Trainees, particularly at the start of their experience with training patients, may sometimes feel overwhelmed with the dynamic processes that abound. They may defend against their anxieties by not being aware of the primitive processes alive in the session or may become so anxious that they cannot articulate what is happening. The supervisor, by contrast, should contain those same primitive processes and through dialogue can establish for the trainee a containing parental couple who can together think about the patient. Both the trainee and the patient experience, through the triangulation of supervision, a good containing parental couple able to work within the Oedipal situation of the supervisory dynamic.

TRAINING: SUPERVISION AND THE THERAPEUTIC FRAME

In therapy, two constants require careful management: one is a process; the other is a non-process, which itself is made up of constants within whose bounds the process takes place. The non-process comprises the frame in which the two people interact and in which the encounter between therapist and patient takes place (Bleger 1967). The frame refers to a strategy rather than a technique: the patient–analyst contract may be understood as an 'agreement between two people into which enter two formal elements of mutual exchange' (Liberman in Bleger 1967: 511) that can confirm the contract, that is time and money. The constants of the frame may, however, trigger and repeat an individual's primitive object-relations, and frame-related issues may activate the primitive process of non-differentiation. This dynamic may be experienced by the patient and the trainee therapist alike and generate powerful transference issues for all participants. One may therefore view the psychotherapeutic situation as a relationship between therapist and patient so that there is a process which is studied, analysed and interpreted.

The therapeutic frame, when thought about in terms of an undifferentiated state (Little 1986), evokes an 'acting in' tendency of the more psychotic parts of the personality and represents a different form of object relatedness. The frame, therefore, may be understood as a permanent presence that replicates the parent for the child, and from this one may infer how any break of the frame, when holidays or unplanned cancellations occur, can be experienced by the patient as a catastrophic situation. 'It is through the detailed work of mourning that differentiation between the self and object are seen more realistically, and the previously disowned parts of the self are gradually acknowledged as belonging to the self' (Steiner 1996: 1077). As such, any deviation in the therapeutic frame can only be understood within the context of the analytic hour. 'In this way the mourning process is replicated in the therapy when the therapist is experienced as separate and independent from the patient who has to face the reality of giving up possessive control over him' (Steiner 1996: 1077).

The same constants apply and operate in supervision as they do in therapy. It is understood, therefore, that the initial frame of supervision, which is the same for both trainees and experienced practitioners, needs to be clearly set up and adhered to, for it is felt that any deviation from that, such as haphazard arrangements or changed appointments, can create anxieties (Langs 1994). The keeping of the frame has a static and a mobile aspect; that is, that supervision is a system, with a process and a non-process, and the supervisory hour parallels the primitive processes implicit in the therapeutic encounter. The supervisor maintains an analytic stance of neutrality while being subjectively and object-ively involved in the material of the work. 'Dynamic factors are always present in the supervisory system and can influence the learning and teaching process for the trainee and the practitioner. It is possible for the trainee to learn and the experienced practitioner to expand upon understanding, in an atmosphere where the analytic frame is observed, and the complexities of boundaries, frame and position are kept clear' (Szecsödy 1990: 260).

Training, therefore, demands of the trainee certain requirements with regard to the therapeutic frame. Many trainings require trainees to see patients with-in external placements. Often supervision is also external, but linked to the training, and sometimes there is additional supervision provided by the train-ing body. The requirements for tape-recordings of sessions or detailed notes and reports might be the demand of the training rather than the placement, and the needs of the trainee may not exactly match the needs of the placement. In rela-tion to the overall frame of the clinical work and training requirements, the organizational and interpersonal dynamics within supervision will be complex.

For example, a GP practice took trainees on placement in order to provide more ongoing therapy and counselling for their patients. A psychotherapist employed by the practice provided supervision. The training organization used the GP practice as a placement for its trainees in order that the trainees could gain a range of experience within a medical setting.

Within the inter-organizational dynamics, a number of factors that required clarification became apparent. The training organization expect-ed that the supervision within the GP practice would provide theoretical input that would enable the trainee to develop their clinical understand-ing. However, the GP practice and their supervisor anticipated that the training had provided the theory and that they would be receiving trainees who had an understanding of clinical work and who could link theory to practice. This was the first split in this interactive dynamic.

Secondly, the trainee was expecting input and assessment from the supervisor in the placement, but this had not been clarified by the train-ing organization. In addition, the trainee anticipated that the patients who were referred would be suitable 'training patients'. The supervisor at the placement had expectations that the trainee would understand issues relating to patient assessment and would be clinically competent. It was clear that each party in this dynamic projected onto the other assumptions and expectations, and that the needs and requirements of each remained undefined.

The danger in such a scenario is that primitive splits and projections lead to blame and recrimination between training and placement, training and trainee, trainee and placement, or placement and trainee, and that this leads to either a breakdown of the process or a failure to learn. It was important in this instance for the supervisor to have a clear contract with the training body, the training body to have a clear contract with the placement and an understanding of the realities and limitations of what is offered, and for both to be explicit about the learning needs of the supervisee. In the above example, the training/supervisory frame had to be understood in terms of the assessment of the needs of the placement and the needs of the trainee so that the needs of the patient could be maintained. The tension within a training can be that the requirements of the training in terms of placements, tape-recorded sessions etc. will eclipse the needs of the patient. When this occurs, the trainee may 'learn' how to be a 'good student' and fulfil the criteria but may not learn how to be a good clinical practitioner whose primary orientation is in understanding the patient.

Training therefore requires that trainees have the space to critically reflect upon their therapeutic work with their training patients within the confines of their training organization or their training supervision. It is often a requirement of the training that process notes and tape-recordings of sessions are kept and used for the purpose of learning within the training supervision. Assumptions about the validity of process notes as a truth about psychic reality and an assessment of a trainee's capability as a practitioner are not without their flaws. And, while a taped session may be presumed to be a more objective record, it too has its limitations as a psychic truth or a clinical fact about a session (see Yorke, chapter 3 of this book). The atmosphere created within the session and what was not said is more likely to be conveyed through the interaction of the supervisor and the supervisee than through the use of the 'objective' tape. 'It is equally difficult in reporting fragments of case material in supervision to convey acting out, which after all one only intuits from the effect that the patient's words produce on the trainee and the atmosphere that is created' (Joseph 1975: 77).

However, just because there are difficulties in attaining objectivity, it should not rule out the continuous need to struggle with bringing to awareness a psychic truth, a clinical fact or a spontaneous gesture. The trainee needs to be familiar with the importance of understanding the here-and-now transference dynamic as it evolves in the therapeutic hour, as well as the constant working through of the ongoing transference dynamic with the patient. These transference interpretations of material presented by the patient are subjectively understood by both the trainee and patient and, indeed, stand as a clinical fact of the moment-to-moment experience within the therapy. When worked with in supervision, it is the moment-to-moment interaction of the transference epitomized in the gesture of the patient, and described by the trainee to the supervisor that is an example of object relationship. Within supervision, and because of its subjective nature, 'a new view of a clinical fact must, like the first one, be subject to validation, as being a truth about the immediate emotional reality between trainee and supervisor' (O'Shaughnessy 1994: 45). This, coupled with the constant monitoring and making sense of countertransference reactions to the material as it presents itself to the trainee is a central task of any supervision, whether training or collegiate. Training practice and supervision causally creates anxieties for the trainee and, to a lesser extent, the experienced practitioner, as they imagine that their newly formulated method of working is under scrutiny. How the trainee makes sense of such imagined scrutiny will depend to some extent on their own psychopathology and the ways in which their training therapy has assisted them in recognizing their own internal object relations.

TRAINING: THE FACILITATING ENVIRONMENT AND SUPERVISION

The trainee, therefore, has to contend with the demands of the training institute and the demands of the patient, a situation in which splitting and projective mechanisms can easily be generated in relation to a phantasy of a 'critical and unloving' training organization and a concomitant defensive and protective reaction to the patient. This paranoid–schizoid dynamic between the training body and the patient, while it remains unconscious, will get played out in supervision, and it is this that the supervisor will need to hold, manage and interpret in a manner which does not confirm the splits that the trainee is caught up in.

While it is acknowledged that in all circumstances patients are of ultimate importance, and their safety and mental welfare have first priority, what is meant by clinical responsibility and where this rests can be an area of conflict between what the training organization, the course leader, the supervisor, as well as the trainee understand this to be. A consequence of this conflict may result in an institutional splitting or schism. However the dynamics are played out, the supervisor has a particular role to play in the holding of the trainee and the training patients.

The tendencies of some training organizations to pathologize their trainees in an attempt to avoid the painful task of raising questions about the efficacy of their training programme is anecdotally only too well known. A defensive training programme will produce defensive training practitioners rather than those who are able or willing to confront the deepest layers of their unconscious. The good-enough training programme is one that is open to acknowledging in its structure that training committees have emotional and psychological needs too. This highlights questions about how best these needs can be served to obtain a good-enough facilitating environment for both the trainee and the trainers within training organizations. Creating a good-enough facilitating environment for the tripartite system of training therapy, theoretical input and supervision can create an interdependent linking of a belief system that is mutually supportive of each faculty. Conversely, any emotional deprivation of an organization can foster each faculty's need to function in an isolated manner, defensively organized to preserve their individuality.

Similarly, it may be believed that the success of a training and a training organization depends upon allegiance to a particular person; a trainer, or therapist, or supervisor so that anxieties are always projected away from the organization itself. Primitive anxieties create cultural pressures that can emanate from the group task within the training organization, and these unconscious collusive forces may permeate and effect relationships with other colleagues. The group and training organization can unconsciously exert control over individual members, and, despite the group's being simultaneously engaged in a joint task, it may also be defending against unconscious anxieties and manipulating the process in the service of defensive needs (Bion 1962).

In a mutually supporting system, contained within a mutually facilitating environment, the supervisor may represent for the trainee a transformational object. Like Winnicott's (1971) concept of the facilitating environment, it may be hoped that the training organizations and supervisors will be able to create good-enough environmental provision at the very earliest stages of the trainee's training for the trainee but also for themselves so that, like the trainee who must relinquish a phantasy of omnipotence, they defer to a mutually supporting system. In this way, the implicit use of transitional phenomena can create an appropriate holding environment for the loss of omnipotence experienced by trainee and training organization alike, which leads to a maturity and the depressive position for both.

The continuity of care has become the central feature of the concept of a facilitating environment. 'A good enough facilitating environment which at the start of each individual's growth and development is a sin qua non' (Winnicott 1971: 163) is as important to the infant at the start of life as it is to the trainee at the start of their training within a training organization. What might be agreed upon as a good-enough facilitating environment for the trainee and trainers may have evolved in design out of unconscious anxieties as to what constitutes appropriate standards of care, and may produce a defensive and rigid model of training. Repressed injuries and hurt to the individual may surface as defensive mechanisms developed to protect against future narcissistic injury, and, paradoxically, narcissistic organizations are often deployed as a defence against pre-Oedipal anxieties. These defensive primitive processes will mitigate against the development of authenticity and creativity within the trainee, and any development, in a defensive environment, may depend upon more than the requirements of the training institute.

Trainees can learn the more technical functions, such as the acquisition of theory or knowledge of psychopathology, where the drive to authenticity dominates the spontaneous gesture. It is here that theoretical instruction and supervision play a role in training. Supervisors are aware that some trainees, while able to learn a great deal of technical expertise and psychodynamic understanding through supervision, may be relatively less able to function sensitively in their capacity to be with their patients. This may continue, even where every effort is made in supervision, to increase the trainee's sensitivity to their own as well as their patient's inner psychic experience (Wolff 1971). To be open to another's emotional reality and to their psychic pain may only be possible if the trainee is familiar with these primitive processes within the self. 'The ability to be with one's patients to a large extent depends on the therapist's own personal characteristics; it clearly demands a considerable degree of empathy and sensitivity to other people's problems and their subjective experience' (Wolff 1971: 128).

The following case illustrates some of these conflicts.

A trainee brought to supervision an emotionally vulnerable young woman whose projective identifications and unconscious demands were continuously overwhelming him. The trainee also brought to supervision issues in terms of training and the way that demands were placed on trainees in relation to note-taking, the collection of fees etc., which the trainee felt were unreasonable and represented an uncaring and persecutory training authority figure, which he felt prevented him from working effectively with the patient.

The supervisor was also aware of the impact of these demands on the clinical work and how they brought 'demands for activity' into the supervisory arena. When the trainee presented the patient, it became apparent that the more the patient operated via splits within the paranoid–schizoid position, the more the trainee moved to a practical and intellectual position in response to his belief that the patient was rapidly fragmenting. The trainee seemed to lose his ability to remain as a therapist and spoke of contacting the patient's medical team, with whom he had ready access.

In exploring the dynamics, the supervisor was able to reflect on how the anxiety created by the patient and her vulnerability seemed to create a resonance that the only way that care could be achieved was via explicit action and expression. The trainee was able to reflect on how the unconscious communication from the patient resonated with his own history of abandonment and abuse and that he was enacting a desire for a loving, reliable and protective parental object through his practical behaviour. As the supervision examined the support system that was in place for this young woman, it became clear to the trainee that the best help that he could offer his patient was to remain firmly situated within the boundaries as her therapist and contain the patient's primitive processes and unconscious demands within the dynamics of the therapy.

Reflecting on this example makes it clear not only that the trainee was expressing some of his own conflicts with the training organization through the patient's material that he was presenting but also that this conflict was affecting the manner in which he was responding to the patient. In his anxiety, he tended to resort to intellectualization and activity. It required the facilitating containment of the supervisor to enable the trainee to be open to a consideration of process and to hold the anxiety and the 'not-knowing' in relation to the patient. The frame of any training, therefore, contains the needs and vulnerabilities of the trainee as well as the needs and vulnerabilities of the patients, and within training these two sets of needs can overlap and conflate and generate defensive reactions that impinge learning. The supervisor, within a training, therefore holds a key facilitative function in the training of a supervisee and their development of understanding and insight about the patient.

TRAINING: SUPERVISION AND THEORY

Until theory and practice begin to become formulated and internalized as a model, the trainee is sometimes lost and confused about their patient's internal object relations and must rely upon prescriptive and reductive intellectualizations about dynamic processes. How to make and understand a dynamic formulation of the patient, which can be gleaned from an enquiry into the historical background and family dynamics of the patient, perhaps becomes more accessible as the trainee begins to develop a confidence in his or her skills as a practitioner. Every practitioner who listens to the biographical data of the patient has to organize what he or she hears into a structure that needs to be kept in mind throughout the therapy. The difficulty for the trainee is how to keep in mind the dynamic formulation and not lose sight of it while working from moment to moment so that each detail has significance in understanding the general map of the patient's internal world. Bion (1962) advocates that the practitioner should appear to approach each session without memory or desire, and Freud (1912) had already recommended the same basic approach when encouraging abstinence, the practice of evenly suspended attention and the bending of one's own unconscious to the patient's.

Within the discipline of psychodynamic training, trainees gradually begin to associate themselves to a particular orientation. Their affiliation to a particular modality may be as much about an unconscious fit between the modality and the trainee as it is about the dyadic experience that evolves between the trainee and the training therapy and/or trainee and training supervision. From a psychodynamic orientation, the trainee has many elements to experience, to understand from a theoretical perspective and to hold for the patient. For instance, the trainee learns how to think causally and historically about their patient, while also working with unconscious processes of splitting and projective identification, or those multifaceted defence mechanisms of regression, denial, idealization, denigration or a flight to a phantasy of repairing the other as a damaged object. For the trainee, these are the building blocks that form the internalized model, and in supervision the trainee is encouraged to maintain hovering attention to these primitive processes.

In training and supervision, the trainee learns that the thrust of an analytic attitude is in the bringing to conscious awareness transference and countertransference communications and how to contain them. The trainee also learns how to manage projective identifications and their possible enactments, and always works in pursuit of understanding and translating symbolic meaning. In supervision, encouragement is given to self enquiry and what Bion (1962) calls a meditative review of clinical work. However, supervision may also become the inevitable place where the trainee's and practitioner's anxieties about not knowing can surface. Anxieties about exposure of this psychic state may be superimposed on the ego's wish for omnipotence; in this way, interpretations that seek to know the ultimate truth make severe demands upon the trainee's functioning superego. In the superego's concern for the welfare of the patient, for whom the trainee or practitioner has clinical responsibility, a particular danger may arise out of the, not infrequent, union between the intellectual approach and a 'false self' (Winnicott 1960) object relationship. When a false self becomes organized in a trainee or experienced practitioner 'who has a high intellectual potential, there is a strong tendency for the mind to become the location for the false self, and in this case there develops a dissociation between intellectual activity and psychosomatic existence' (Winnicott 1960: 144).

A trainee may develop an undue emphasis on theory, the need to know and conscious and rational reality, because the capacity to live with the not knowing and the irrational experiences of human reality is too difficult. Where the trainer or supervisor has not been able to stimulate within the trainee the capacity to play with an interpretation, or to encourage free associations, a resistance is present and a regression to concrete thinking or omnipotent intellectualization will develop. Omnipotent intellectualization unconsciously operates to keep the unknown and needy parts of the self hidden, and prevents that needy part from ever being understood. Winnicott points out that there is a danger when there is a 'tie-up between the intellectual approach and the false self' (Winnicott 1960: 144) and that when an individual attempts to 'solve personal problems by the use of a fine intellect, a clinical picture results, which is peculiar in that it very easily deceives' (Winnicott 1960: 144). This intellectualization may deceive both the training organization and the supervisor, who may collude with this pseudo intellect. 'The world may observe academic success of a high degree, and may find it hard to believe in the very real distress of the individual concerned, who feels phoney the more he is successful' (Winnicott 1960: 144). The organized false self, and a defensive intellectualization, may create an intellectual and academic understanding of theory, and yet it reflects a rigidity of defence that prevents any true growth and development within the trainee. This presents something of a paradox within supervision, during training and afterwards because practitioners need analytic thinking to inform their work, but they also need to heed that moment when that same informed thinking interferes with the capacity to listen to what the patient is saying (Steiner 1996).

Although theory and a body of knowledge is a requirement of any training, one of the primary factors which a trainee needs to appreciate is that they must often rely upon themselves as a tool of the work. What is internal and what is external reality becomes the key issue so that the task of supervision is one of encouragement and helping the trainee to understand the value of just being there for the patient, while nurturing their ability to contain their patient's anxieties and primitive processes and understand the unconscious communications. In this sense, the supervisor becomes the container for the trainee's new experiences of processing the primitive paranoid-schizoid states of their patients and offers to them a model of an analytic attitude and reflective stance.

Bion (1962) places the capacity to know at the centre of mental life and argues that the origins of thinking evolved out of those primitive communications projected into the mother for her to know and to process. In supervision, the trainee unravels projective identifications and learns from those emotional experiences with the supervisor. This means that the trainee must notice them, understand their nature and remember them: that is to think. Failure to use the emotional experiences produces a comparable disaster in the development of the personality (Bion 1962). Initially, the trainee may want to regress to a somewhat cocooned state during supervision; however, the supervisor's task is to keep the 'third object', the patient, in mind – thus preventing supervision becoming therapy. In this way, the Oedipal situation that marks a maturity in thinking and knowing becomes a part of an internalized structure of an analytic body of knowledge within the supervisee.

For example, a recent graduate of a psychodynamic training was in a transitional stage from trainee to professional practitioner and was struggling to let go of his training supervision to find his own style. He brought to supervision a young man who was hard to reach, despite the creative work that was implicit in the therapy. It was apparent in the supervisee's presentations that a negative transference was dominant and that the supervisee consciously felt abused by his patient, hopeless about the task and anxious that he could not hold the patient during the working through of the paranoid–schizoid anxieties.

The supervisor was aware that the supervisee was re-experiencing the disorientation of being a beginner within this new and transitional phase of becoming an independent practitioner. The completion of training, and the struggle with the patient, brought to the fore issues around limitations and the mourning of the lost, idealized internal or external object that the training and being a trainee had represented. As such, the supervisee was struggling with the transition to a depressive position in relation to his clinical work and his view of himself as a professional practitioner. In focusing on the work with the patient, the supervisor was aware that the issues which the patient was bringing reflected anger at the failure of the idealized therapist. The supervisor also identified that the struggle within the work was to contain the anxieties of both the therapist and the patient. The supervisor was aware that these anxieties needed to be held so that the transference and counter-transference dynamics could be considered, and the defences and projections explored, in relation to the patient's internal world, and that this exploration would enable a working through of the paranoid-schizoid splits, projections and defences.

Trainees will inevitably project onto a training internal-world issues in much the same way that a patient projects their hopes, phantasies and internal objects onto the therapist. Training therefore impacts on the internal world of the trainee, and so internal motifs will be activated. Those that resonate with the supervisee's anxieties will be reflected in the supervision (Searles 1955). The supervisor, therefore, needs to maintain the focus on the supervisory task while remaining mindful of the developmental needs of the trainee. In the example above, both the patient and the supervisee were struggling with the holding of opposites and the dimensions of disillusionment. For the supervisee, this also involved issues of separation and loss and the Oedipal situation as he struggled towards maturity. It was only when the issues could be separated out and the reflection process (Searles 1955) be understood that the supervisee could understand the issues that the patient was unconsciously communicating. In

the processing of this experience, both supervisee and supervisor had to consider how the supervisee was a 'tool' in relation to the patient's communication
and that the resonance of the internal-world issues between supervisee and
patient provided a medium through which the patient's unconscious struggles
were communicated. Developing an understanding and insight into this
requires a combination of theory and reflection, understanding and emotional
processing in a dialectic in which theory alone would not have been sufficient.

TRAINING: COUNTERTRANSFERENCE CONSIDERATIONS AND SUPERVISION

Trainees are often confused about their reactions to their patients and often
interpret their reactions as something emotionally aberrant within their own
mental processes. The significance given to countertransference and the importance attached to the corresponding problems depends upon the significance
given to the role of the therapist. From a psychodynamic perspective, both the
trainee and the professional practitioner are interpreters of unconscious processes, and the objects of those same processes. In supervision the unpacking of the
countertransference is instrumental in bringing to the trainee's attention a psychological fact about the patient. The danger, especially for an inexperienced
practitioner, is of 'acting out' in relation to countertransference or of acting in a
retaliatory manner in relation to perceived conscious or unconscious 'attacks'
from the patient. Racker describes this in terms of talion law and writes, 'every
positive transference situation is answered by a positive countertransference'
(Racker 1991: 137), and every negative transference is responded to on the part
of the therapist by a negative countertransference. It is a helpful concept because
a conscious awareness of talion law is fundamental in the sense that it avoids the
trainee drowning in the countertransference and acting out in a retaliatory manner towards the patient. 'Failure to be aware of the inevitable pitfalls of this
dynamic will lead to entering into the vicious circle of the patient's neurosis and
will hinder or prevent the work of the therapy' (Racker 1991: 137).

It was Heimann (1950) who showed how the use of countertransference was
an important tool for understanding the patient, provided it could be differentiated from pathological countertransference responses. Later, Searles (1955)
made the important link between the supervisor's emotional experience – his
countertransference – and the patient's unconscious communications via the
reflection process. For Racker (1991), it is understood that the transference and
countertransference represents two components of a unity mutually giving life
to each other and creating the interpersonal relationship of the analytic situation. Heimann (1950) shows that unconscious phantasy, in which the therapist

is involved, means that, whether the transference interpretation was tentative or forthright, it was always attempting to address what was happening in the here and now of the clinical setting. This differentiation, which was an important development in thinking about unconscious processes, is essential, within the clinical reality, for there is no such thing as absolute separation between transference and countertransference phenomena, only relative movement within that orbit. 'The point is that we have to cope with feelings and subject them to thought for we are not neutral in the sense of having no reactions to the work' (Brenman Pick 1985: 41).

Using oneself as a tool and understanding the interplay between countertransference and transference is vital in the development of clinical work and learning within the trainee. Problems arise when supervisees are unable to process experience. 'Errors in technique very often reflect a failure on the part of the psychotherapist to process adequately the patient's projective identifications, perhaps through denial, splitting, and other projective mechanisms' (Ogden 1979: 368). This defensive stance may be paralleled within the supervision. The trainee needs to bring all emotional experiences of the therapy into supervision, and failure to do so may result in dire consequences for the progress of the clinical work.

In supervision, the trainee needs to be encouraged to work through such experiences, perhaps feeling like an overwhelmed mother threatened with disintegration by an overwhelming baby. These are situations that are best managed with the supervisor as representative of the third object to support the clinical experience within a facilitating environment. Understanding and working with countertransference reactions becomes clearer for the more experienced practitioner as there develops a qualitative shift from external transference figures brought by the patient as representations of their internal worlds to experiencing what is apparent in the here and now of object relations. Observed and imaginative events take place in a world conceived of as contiguous in time and space and given structure by Oedipal configurations. 'It includes, therefore, the possibility of being a participant in a relationship and observed by a third person, as well as being an observer of a relationship between two people' (Britton 1989: 86).

CONCLUSION

In the present climate of transparency, tensions can surface as to what should be open to public scrutiny and what remain confidential. This is also pertinent to training organizations and concerns the issue of whether training assessments can be open and seen by all trainees or closed and secretive. The latter mode encourages secretiveness, replicates the Oedipal situation of exclusion and the phantasies of what goes on behind closed doors. Likewise, dependence upon one's trainer, if unresolved, can replicate the Oedipal situation and maintain a transference dynamic that is never resolved. Change has to arise from within and depends upon a capacity to think and judge for oneself so that developmentally for the trainee it involves 'a relinquishment of a dependence on the views and judgements of authority figures, including the training therapist, supervisor, and training organisation' (Steiner 1996: 1076). Similarly, Racker comments, 'real independence would be based upon the trainee depending upon an internal object that neither imposes nor threatens but loves, accepting or refusing without fear or hatred. This internal object relationship determines the relations to external objects' (Racker 1991: 182).

Unconscious processes are powerful and can subvert the positive conscious goals and planning of training programmes so that training organizations may regress or individuals split off into subgroups where eventual disintegration may occur. The aims and objectives of training programmes need to be clearly agreed upon and administered, while acknowledgement be given to how external and internal developmental needs and ethical requirements coalesce and result in appropriate change. 'There may be a sense that the educational process of psychoanalytic training today may be conducted in an atmosphere of indoctrination rather than scientific enquiry, and that this creates a flatness in educational style, where there is a lack of sharing of analytic experience with students, and where analytic orthodoxy is the institution' (Kernberg 1986: 799). Where benign superego dynamics operate to condition the trainee's sense of their own integrity as a psychotherapist within a training, the trainee will be able to use the here and now to critically engage with the content and process of the experience. The important focus for any supervision must be to encourage trainees to listen to their own countertransference reactions and for the supervisor to affirm their trainee's integrity as therapist. 'Patients touch off in the analyst deep issues and anxieties related to the need to be loved and the fear of catastrophic consequences in the face of defects, such as primitive persecutory or superego anxiety' (Brenman Pick 1985: 41). These primitive processes may be touched off within the training organization eager to support its trainees through training but lacking a strong sense of its own ethical integrity as an institution.

In this chapter, I have attempted to open up for discussion my pivotal question as to whether the art of psychotherapy, which is born out of a complex system of interrelated theoretical elements, is innate within the trainee and professional practitioner or developed through training, learning and supervision. It is clear that the trainee, having been selected for training, stands in one position, the training organization stands at another, the trainer at another and the supervisor at another. Each has their own expectations, hopes and idealizations about this developmental journey, and each consciously and unconsciously exerts pressure upon the other to control the outcome. Perhaps the making of a good-enough therapist is more about how much they can bring of themselves to the task of the work than what theoretical model they have internalized. Whichever that may be, what is wished for is that the trainee, through sensitive interactions within this complex system, develops within the orbit of a good-enough facilitating environment and maturationally moves from a paranoid-schizoid position to the depressive position and psychological maturity.

REFERENCES

Balint M (1948) On the psychoanalytic training system. International Journal of Psycho-Analysis 29(1-2): 163–173.

Bion WR (1962) A theory of thinking. International Journal of Psycho-Analysis 43(4-5): 649–657.

Bleger J (1967) Psycho-analysis of the psycho-analytic frame. International Journal of Psycho-Analysis 48(4): 511–519.

Brenman Pick I (1985) Working through in the countertransference. In Bott Spillius E (ed.) (1994) Melanie Klein Today: Developments in theory and practice. Volume 2: Mainly Practice. London and New York: Routledge.

Britton R (1989) 'The missing link'. In Britton R, Feldman M, O'Shaughnessy E (eds), The Oedipus Complex Today: Clinical Implications. London: Karnac Books.

Driver C (2002) Internal States in the Supervisory Relationship. In Driver C, Martin E (eds) Supervising Psychotherapy. London: Sage Publications.

Driver C, Martin E (2002) Supervising Psychotherapy: Psychoanalytic and Psychodynamic Perspectives. London: Sage Publications.

Freud S (1909) 'The third lecture'. In Strachey J (ed.), (1962) Two Short Accounts of Psycho-Analysis. Harmondsworth: Penguin Books.

Freud S (1912) Recommendations To Physicians Practicing Psycho-Analysis. SE 12. London: Hogarth Press.

Hawkins P, Shohet R (2002) Supervision in the Helping Professions. Buckingham: Open University Press.

Heimann P (1950) On counter-transference. International Journal of Psycho-Analysis 31(1): 81–84.

Joseph B (1975) 'The patient who is hard to reach'. In Bott Spillius E, Feldman M (eds) (1989), Psychic Equilibrium and Psychic Change: Selected Papers of Betty Joseph. London: Routledge.

Kernberg, O. (1986) Institutional problems of psycho-analytic education. Journal of American Psycho-Analysis 34(4): 799–834.

Klein M (1930) 'The importance of symbol formation'. In Mitchell J (ed.) (1986), The Development of the Ego. The Selected Melanie Klein. London: Hogarth Press.

Langs R (1994) Doing Supervision and Being Supervised. London: Karnac Books.

Little M (1986) 'On basic unity: primary total undifferentiatedness'. In Kohon G (ed.), The British School of Psychoanalysis: The Independent Tradition. London: Free Association Books.

Lloyd-Owen D (2003) Perverse females: their unique pathology. British Journal of
    Psychotherapy 19(3): 285–296.
Ogden TH (1979) On projective identification. International Journal of Psycho-Analysis 60(2):
    357–373.
O'Shaughnessy E (1981) A commemorative essay on WR Bion's *Theory Of Thinking*. Journal of
    Child Psychotherapy 7(2): 181–189.
O'Shaughnessy E (1994) 'What is a clinical fact?' In Schafer R (ed.) (1997), The Contemporary
    Kleinians of London. Madison, CT: International University Press.
Racker T (1991) Transference And Counter-Transference. London: Karnac Books.
Roustang, F. (1982) Drive Mastery. Baltimore: Johns Hopkins University Press.
Searles HF (1955) 'The information value of the supervisor's emotional experiences'. In Searles
    HF (1986), Collected Papers on Schizophrenia and Related Subjects. London: Maresfield
    Library.
Segal H (1986) Delusion and Artistic Creativity and other Psychoanalytic Essays. London: Free
    Association Books.
Steiner J (1996) The aim of psychoanalysis in theory and practice. International Journal of
    Psycho-Analysis 77(6): 1073–1083.
Szecsödy I (1990) Supervision: a didactic or mutative experience. Psychoanalytic
    Psychotherapy 4(3): 245–261.
Thomas S (1997) Supervision as a maturational process. Psychodynamic Counselling 3(1): 63–76.
Winnicott WD (1956) 'On transference'. In Esman AH (ed.) (1990), Essential Papers on
    Transference. New York: University Press.
Winnicott WD (1960) 'Ego distortion in terms of the true and false self'. In The Maturational
    Process and the Facilitating Environment (1990). London: Karnac Books.
Winnicott WD (1971) Playing And Reality. Harmondsworth and New York: Penguin Books.
Wolff, H. (1971) The therapeutic and developmental function of psychotherapy. British
    Medical Journal of Psychiatry 44(1): 117–128.

CHAPTER 10

SUPERVISION: ETHICAL PRACTICE AND THE LAW

RUTH BARNETT

INTRODUCTION

There is much fear surrounding supervisors and therapists being caught in litigation and how therapeutic language may be misconstrued in the legal process. Are lawyers friends or enemies, and how can legal and therapeutic languages meet? This chapter will explore some ways the therapy profession has responded to contextual changes in society. The supervisory role in ethical practice, especially in relation to disclosure to a third party and issues of clinical responsibility, has become increasingly important. Good intentions are not enough for good practice. Today's therapists must hone their skills with continuous professional development, supervision and other reflective dialogue.

WHAT IS ETHICAL PRACTICE?

An example can show the need to address this issue. In February 2001, the *London Review of Books* published an article by Wynne Godley, 'Saving Masud Khan' (Godley 2001), telling the story of Godley's long analysis with Khan, a psychoanalyst who was greatly revered professionally. During his analysis, Godley had suffered extreme verbal abuse, anxiety and humiliation at the hands of Khan, who broke every conceivable boundary. Yet, other analysands benefited greatly from their analyses with Khan and some went on to become notable analysts themselves. Khan 'the sadist and torturer' with Godley was a 'gentle genius' with others.

Why did a highly trained and effective healer harm some of his patients? Who was responsible? The seducer, the overly trusting victim or the colluding bystanders? Damage to the vulnerable patient might have been curtailed if colleagues in a position to do so had taken action on what they knew or suspected. Khan was the protégé of two eminent analysts at the time, Donald Winnicott and Anna Freud, and, no doubt, it would have been daunting for any of those aware of the abuse to act. Furthermore, Winnicott himself broke boundaries flagrantly where Khan was concerned.

This is an example of clearly unethical practice that did not come to light until all the main protagonists of the drama except the victim were dead. Many perpetrators of professional abuse, misconduct and malpractice continue to act out their abusive fantasies today in a fog of secrecy and cruelty while those in the know prevaricate and are paralysed to act. Opportunities for power differential between vulnerable needy patients and narcissistic power-hungry professionals are unavoidable. Freud is purported to have said that without the power to do harm you cannot have the power to do good either.

This cannot be used as an excuse to evade professional responsibility. In the past, roles like 'doctor' or 'parent' were revered, and, if abuse came to light at all, the victim was blamed. Evasion of responsibility and sacrifice of ethical principles in the service of protecting idealized institutions undoubtedly contributed to the impunity with which Khan was able to perpetrate abuse. Today, values and morals have changed substantially. Reverence has evaporated, trust and esteem have to be earned and patients are now more worldly wise and psychologically sophisticated. Many of even the most eminent therapists of 50 years ago would be found wanting if judged by today's more rigorous standards. Supervision has gradually acquired an ever more central and responsible role in the provision of mental health services. Training to supervise is increasingly expected as supervision is becoming recognized as more than just an extension of experienced practice. There is even a tendency to expect supervisors to take on a false role as guardians of professional responsibility. The therapy profession needs supervisors who are both thoroughly conversant with ethical practice and also able to engender its development in their supervisees.

Ethical codes, mandatory for membership of all the main therapy organizations, no longer have the relevance they had at first. They proved unable to replace the old reliance on appointed authorities who carried the can for everything as they could not prescribe for every complex situation. The essence of therapy and supervision is process. There can be no absolutes. Prescriptive codes have served us in the interim and are giving way now to guidelines and principles for taking responsibility at an individual practitioner level. Supervision plays an essential role in a profession that is continually developing.

THE ROLE OF THE LAW

The evolution of society's values precipitates review and new laws to respond to change. Therapists do not usually become lawyers, and most lawyers do not have much opportunity to experience or appreciate the principles on which therapy is based. This creates a potential for misrepresentation and misunderstanding when therapists or their organizations become involved in litigation. Rules of law that are intended to achieve justice may clash with basic tenets of essential importance to therapists. For example, they differ regarding the circumstances in which confidential material can be disclosed. This has caused anxiety among those therapists who perceive the law as threatening to damage their profession. Likewise, some lawyers regard therapists as secretive, uncooperative or challenging their prerogatives. Misunderstanding can lead to hostility that is likely to be detrimental to both therapists and lawyers. Lawyers draw on arguments and judgments that have been made in past cases, and recent Acts have not yet been proven in this respect. Much anxiety is fuelled by the fear that this system of case law might develop to the detriment of the therapy profession. This need not be so. The majority of lawyers and therapists respect their clients' vulnerabilities and do not prey on them. Ethical practice requires therapists to understand the recent changes in the law that have a bearing on their profession.

Training courses have neglected this area in the past, when litigation involving therapists was rare, but are starting to respond to this need, and therapy organizations encourage continuing professional development (CPD) units on ethical practice and law. Supervisors may find themselves in the forefront of these changes as more supervisees become directly involved with litigation or have to make difficult professional decisions that might lead to brushes with the law. For example, as demographics predict a rapid increase in elderly people needing care, supervisees will be seeing patients struggling to cope with elderly relatives as well as children and work. There are likely to be complex issues around stress, neglect, abuse, suicide and even euthanasia.

Several developments in the law are important. The European Convention on Human Rights has compelled reviews of domestic laws, and there are problems when British laws are at variance with those of Brussels. The Access to Personal Files Act of 1987, Medical Records Act of 1988, Children Act of 1989, Access to Health Records Act of 1990 and Data Protection Act of 1998 all need to be taken into account by supervisors regarding the contracts they make with patients, supervisees and therapy agencies. The implications of these laws also affect the decisions to be made. Conflicts between different ethical principles of practice are becoming more frequent, making the reflective work of supervision ever more demanding.

DIFFERENT LANGUAGES: A CASE OF LITIGATION

Therapists may find themselves involved with four languages that can become entangled in litigation. Therapists, lawyers, medical practitioners and ordinary members of the public use certain words that are specific to their own familiar domain and use other words in common but with different shades of meaning. The differences can be subtle and yet lead to gross misunderstandings and failures of communication. An actual case can illustrate this:

> The clinical director of a counselling organization received a letter from a solicitor requesting notes and records of a client's counselling that had ended six years previously and enclosing a form signed by the client giving her permission. The director faced two problems: how to deal with records and notes written by a counsellor no longer in the organization and how to validate the client's consent. In fact, the client's own solicitor had told her that she had to sign or her case would be thrown out. Informed consent had different meanings in the solicitor's and director's languages.
>
> The director found the client's file in the organization's records and arranged to meet with the client to validate it. The client was reluctant and angry that the director would not send the records without a meeting. The client and director were speaking different languages. However, the client appreciated the difference when she met the director to read through the records. She found an error that the director then rectified before she signed a new consent form on the organization's headed paper, which was then sent to the solicitor.
>
> The solicitor was not satisfied with the organizational records and demanded session notes, which he insisted the counsellor must have made, or written verification that the notes had been professionally destroyed. The director contacted the counsellor, who responded, 'Of course I have not destroyed anything – it is all safely locked away.' She established that the counsellor's notes, in hardly readable shorthand, would be of dubious use. She reported this to the solicitor, who ordered that the counsellor type out her notes and submit an expense account. The director negotiated a price with the counsellor, arriving at a sum that she hoped would put the solicitor off. The director and the counsellor then each received a subpoena to appear in court with the notes intact and a cheque for £20. The director, feeling insulted that her time was deemed to be worth only £20, became anxious and angry. The counsellor promptly furnished herself with medical certification that her heart condition would be seriously jeopardized by appearing in court.

The director realized that she might have spared herself and the coun-sellor a lot of anxiety by seeking advice earlier. She had a bare two weeks before the court hearing. The situation seemed to have reached an impasse. How could she disclose the notes in question without informed consent? How could she ask the client to read the session notes to valid-ate them? To whom did the notes belong anyway? They almost certainly contained sensitive information about the client, but about other people too. Might a solicitor reading them misinterpret them? What would this mean for the client? How would it reflect on her own practice, that of the counsellor, her organization and the profession?

Her supervisor questioned the director's contract with the organiza-tion. What was the policy on confidentiality and notes? The director consulted the chairman of the organization, who saw no problem and said, 'Just send the notes. We do it all the time in the NHS.' The direct-or was caught between two professional cultures and could not convince her chairman that counselling notes are sensitive because they are not only confidential but also deal in narrative truth and unconscious processes that can be mistaken for historical truth and reality. She was into yet another conflict. If she obeyed her boss' directive, she would be going against her own ethical principles. She considered the confiden-tial session notes could not help the court to establish truth and might be misinterpreted to the client's detriment. So she did what therapists and supervisors should be advised to do as part of their training or CPD. She set about finding out her options and what the outcome had been for those who already had similar experience. She discovered the £20 cheque was a court formality that had nothing to do with the value of her time. She learnt how solicitors and courts function. She found out what support the organization's indemnity insurers would provide and what limits they would set. She gathered advice and support from the BACP and colleagues. She discovered some therapists had disclosed material in court while others had managed to avoid this. A psychiatrist who was subpoenaed and refused in court to disclose any confidential material of her client's therapy was knowingly in contempt of court and risked prison. The judge respected her courage and integrity and neither required her to disclose nor sent her to prison. Lord Bingham describes this case in an article published in the *British Journal of Psychotherapy* (Bingham 2003).

Acting on information and advice she had collected, some of which was contradictory, the director decided to appeal to the court. With her chairman's agreement, she wrote a careful letter claiming that the nature of the session notes made them vulnerable to misinterpretation by anyone not familiar with unconscious processes. She argued that the notes should be addressed in chambers (client and public not present) with an expert witness to interpret them. Whether her argument was accepted or an expert witness deemed too costly, the subpoena was subsequently withdrawn. The director had been shaken out of her complacency and took responsibility for generating discussions to produce a comprehensive organizational policy on notes and records in line with the Data Protection Act (1998) and the new BACP's *Ethical Framework for Good Practice in Counselling and Psychotherapy* (BACP 2002).

THE DATA PROTECTION ACT

The Data Protection Act is a monster but, like the fairytale *Shrek*, is a friendly one. Nobody is expected to know everything and get everything right all the time. Despite its size, the Act cannot prescribe for every eventuality. It aims to encourage reflection on the use of information about other people and informed responsible decisions on handling data. The worst scenario is that the Data Information Commissioner gets a complaint and is bound by the Act to investigate. The person or organization being investigated needs to demonstrate good practice: honesty, transparency and intent to carry out the principles of the Act. They should be able to answer for what purpose they have collected data and for whose benefit it is held. They should also have policy in place for keeping their data up to date and properly destroying it immediately it has served its purpose.

The Data Protection Act (1998) required organizations to 'register' with the Data Information Commissioner and laid down requirements for registered organizations. The 1998 Act demands compliance with its requirements for processing 'personal data' by individuals as well as organizations, whether they are required or exempt from having to 'notify' the Information Commissioner. The Act defines personal data as any information about 'identifiable living individuals' in a manual or computer system structured for easy access including anything (post, in-tray, emails) that will go into the systems. 'Data processing' means collecting, holding, storing, altering, updating, retrieving, giving out, destroying or doing anything else with personal data. The 'data controller' is the organization or person who collects and files the data and determines its purposes. The data controller sets the policy for how data is to be processed by agents, called the data processors. The data controller carries responsibility for complying with the principles of the Act. Therapists in private practice are their own data controllers and data processors. In agencies, the management team is responsible.

The principles of the Data Protection Act are that data processing must be fair, for designated purposes only, adequate, relevant, up to date and not excessive or continue longer than necessary for its purpose. The rights of data subjects and appropriate security must be ensured. 'Fair processing' means that data subjects are informed about, and sometimes written consent is sought for, what is done with their data. They must not be deceived. 'Sensitive data' includes details of racial origin, beliefs, political opinions, criminal records, health and sexual history (but not financial details) and must be kept particularly secure. 'Data subject rights' means data subjects can ask to see and have a copy of data kept about them. Up to £10 administration fees can be charged for giving the subject a copy. Allowance has to be made for data subjects to opt in or out of certain data processing, where appropriate and reasonable. Giving out lists and advertising are examples of where data subjects should be given the possibility to opt in or out. The emphasis is on 'reasonable'. Consent is needed for what is done with data defined as 'sensitive'. Filling in a form can constitute consent as long as it gives information about what will be done with the data.

If the only personal data kept on computer is 'core business' about members and contacts in agencies, notifying the Information Commissioner (which would mean paying an annual fee and giving details of data kept) is not necessary. To demonstrate 'good intent', an individual or organization needs to review their data-processing purposes and create a clear, written policy stating what personal data are processed, for what purpose(s) and for how long. The data controller needs to make sure the subjects of personal data know their rights.

THE BACP's ETHICAL FRAMEWORK FOR GOOD PRACTICE IN COUNSELLING AND PSYCHOTHERAPY

This document came into force in April 2002. It replaces all former BAC(P) codes of ethics and complaints procedures. A commitment to accepting it is a requirement for BACP membership. This new framework lays down no rules for practice but focuses on principles, responsibilities, values and basic personal qualities for good practice. It includes a new procedure for complaints of unprofessional conduct. The spirit of the *Framework* does not aim for 'perfection' or 'problem-free' practice. It emphasizes the need for counsellors to reflect on what they do and know why they do it. Responsibility includes taking risks, especially when all the options available, including doing nothing, carry some risk. It means knowing what the options are (adequate training and CPD), reflecting on them (adequate supervision and support) and being able to account for the course of action or inaction chosen when it turns out to have unforeseen or untoward consequences. Complainants no longer have to find a 'rule' that the complained against has breached. Instead, if informal procedures have not reached a resolution, they are encouraged to write their grievance in as much detail as possible. A BACP Pre-Hearing Assessment Panel decides whether there is a case to answer, or more information is needed, or there are inadequate grounds for complaint. In the formal procedure, the defendant needs to answer for what they did and why they did it, to demonstrate responsible, reflective practice, decisions and actions in the spirit of the *Framework*.

PROCESS NOTES, CASE STUDIES AND PUBLICATION

Freud was emphatic that psychoanalysts had a responsibility amounting to an obligation to make available what they learnt from their analytic work. How else could colleagues in different parts of the world learn from each other and new analysts get adequate training? Freud's own writings contained meticulous details about his patients. It became a common practice among therapists to include session material in articles and books they published. Usually, the patient's name was altered and other factors, not essential to the process being portrayed, were disguised so that the patient would not be recognized. Cases of patients or relatives recognizing the material were extremely rare, as they were unlikely to attend professional meetings or read psychoanalytic journals and books. This has changed in the last few decades. New therapies have developed and are available to a much broader section of the public. More patients than formerly now read clinical articles and books and some surf the Internet deliberately to find what their therapists have written.

Every aspect of writing about patients, from a jotted *aide-mémoire* to published books, is now under scrutiny. The Data Protection Act requires data subjects to be informed of the purposes for which data about them will be used and their consent obtained. This could be taken to mean that all therapists must inform their patients if they are going to make session notes. If the notes are to be an *aide-mémoire* only, it can be argued that informing the patient should be waived. Perhaps both patient and therapist would be better off if the therapist opts to make no notes at all and simply relies on their memory recall for all situations. This, too, would entail a risk. The therapist might at some time have to face accusations of neglectful practice and need to account for their reasons in making a particular decision and explain the benefit to the patient. Patients have fantasies about whether or not their therapist makes notes about them. A door is closed to exploring these fantasies if the patient is informed. But another door is still open to exploring what the information means to the patient.

The law has a protective role in relation to the individual, the public and the state. The Data Protection Act takes its name from its aim to protect people against any abuse of their personal details. It gives data subjects the right of access at any time to their data to check their accuracy and validity. Patients, therefore, have a right to see any information their therapists hold about them. Usually, if a patient insists on seeing their therapist's notes, it means that trust, and with it the therapeutic alliance, has broken down. Supervision or other consultation could help to decide the way forward. It is not clear whether the notes the therapist makes belong to the patient or the therapist. Are the notes about the patient or about the therapist's experience of the patient? Are they factual data or the therapist's narrative of the patient's narrative? If the notes do not contain the patient's name or other means of identification, it might be argued that the data subject is the 'therapist in their experience of their work' and not the patient they have been working with. Trainee therapists would be deprived of valuable learning potential if they were not allowed to make notes to take to supervision, or to write case studies, without the intrusion of obtaining a patient's consent. Obtaining permission from the patient would inevitably be intrusive and necessitate careful thought about how the intrusion was to be managed. Should the training organization obtain the consent or the trainee? If supervisors make notes, these could be subpoenaed. What kind of evidence such notes might represent needs to be addressed. It might be argued that a supervisor's notes could not be relevant, as they would be the supervisor's narrative of the therapist's narrative of the patient's narrative.

There is an important difference between facts and narrative, which is difficult for both lawyers and therapists to grasp. Whenever serious complications emerge in therapy or there are indications that they might develop, an important factor in handling the situation is for the supervisor and supervisee to disentangle facts from narrative and record as much factual data as possible. It can concentrate the mind for making difficult decisions, and help in accounting for those decisions, if there are careful records of factual developments with dates, decisions made and results of decisions. These are then records as distinguished from process notes.

Writing notes for articles and books intended for publication is a different matter. The general public has become much more psychologically aware and likely to read and recognize patients (or supervisees), even in clinical material that is disguised. Rather than a prescriptive code of practice to ensure that this never happens, the public and the profession are better served by dealing with situations honestly and fairly when they arise.

For example, a supervisee arrived for supervision in a distraught state. Her patient had read an article in a therapy journal and was convinced that her therapist had written it under a pseudonym. He was unable to believe that the clinical vignette in it was not about himself. This is an issue that supervisors need to be prepared to meet and consider how they might work on it with their supervisee.

Let us suppose that the therapist had actually written the article and the clinical material was from the therapy with the patient who had recognized it. She would be acting unethically to deny it. Ethical practice would require her to own it and explore with her patient what it meant to him. Did he feel misrepresented or insulted? What influence might his knowledge of the article have on his therapy and his feelings about his therapist? Would he have preferred his therapist to seek his consent before she wrote about him and would he have given it? The experience might be a damaging one for both patient and therapist, but it also might be an instigator for growth and enrich the therapy. The supervisor has an important role to hold and contain the therapist's anxiety, so that they can reflect together on the options relevant to the situation and the therapist make a considered ethical decision on how to proceed.

There are many complexities requiring clarification in ethical practice before responsible individual decisions can be made. A serious point to debate might be whether there should be mandatory informed consent by the patient for their therapist to make notes or records of sessions, including permission for identified purposes the notes might fulfil. It is interesting to ponder on how this might affect confidentiality and whether this would benefit patients in the long run or not. Patients with problems around trusting would be likely to experience their therapist's seeking consent as intrusive. Session notes can be made unidentifiable and need not be kept very long, perhaps only until used in supervision, before being destroyed. If only notes of a few sessions exist at any time, this would enhance the argument against their constituting patient data. But this would not be possible if notes would be needed for longer-term purposes. The core of the issue is the protection of confidentiality, which itself has to be under scrutiny.

CONFIDENTIALITY

Ethical practice has always required therapists to provide the highest possible levels of confidentiality to respect the patient's privacy and create the trust necessary for a therapeutic alliance. Some people, at least in the past, have interpreted this as implying a need for absolute confidentiality. This has never actually existed, as therapists need to talk about their patients in professional settings, like consultative referral, supervision and seminars. To promise a patient 'absolute confidentiality' is irresponsible and unethical. The most therapists can do is to assure their patients of the highest level of confidentiality consistent with the law and the code of ethics to which they subscribe. How this assurance is to be given, by whom, and at what stage in the process of patients' application and referral for treatment, needs careful consideration. To avoid mention of confidentiality or to dismiss the issue with 'of course our service is confidential', with no further explanation, would be unethical. Repercussions later may show that the patient has misunderstood the boundaries, and the therapist might be accused of unethical practice and neglect. If there were serious implications that led to a professional-conduct process, the therapist would need to demonstrate the thinking behind taking the action or inaction. The argument would have to take into account the tension between the legal obligation for therapists to protect the personal confidences of their clients and the use of their professional judgement to make ethical decisions about confidentiality.

British law concerning confidentiality is evolving. At present, it contains several different approaches to 'legally privileged right to privacy' and 'protection of personal information'. Lord Bingham explains, in his article on confidentiality, the general meaning of what is called by lawyers 'legal professional privilege'. In absolute terms, this applies only to lawyers in relation to their client's confidences. However, it has in fact applied in most situations also to priests with confessional confidences, journalists regarding the identity of their sources and the medical and therapy professions with sensitive patient data. Individual cases centre on what is in the public's interest to be disclosed. There is no clear case law as yet to define how Human Rights laws and the Data Protection Act of 1998 affect legal professional privilege. Solicitors may try to exact the maximum advantage for their own clients, but courts of law and judges tend to protect private confidence unless it can be argued as counter to the public's interest. Since the Woolf Report (Dehn 1995) in 1995, litigation has necessarily become less aggressive. Therapists do not have to comply with requests from solicitors or other people for documents, such as notes or summaries, or demands to appear in court. Only a judge can subpoena a therapist to attend court and/or to produce documents. Refusal to comply with a subpoena constitutes 'contempt of court'. As such, it can warrant a prison sentence. But, even in court, disclosure can and has been refused in certain cases, such as the one described by Lord Bingham (2003).

A therapist who can demonstrate a conscientious decision in the interests of the patient is better placed legally than someone who adopts an inflexible stance or neglects to reflect on all aspects of the specific situation in an issue of confidentiality. Oral evidence of personal recollection (both the patient's and therapist's) is vulnerable to doubt. For this reason, many therapists find a way of giving their patients written information. There are many examples of literature designed to inform patients briefly of what to expect in therapy. The bottom line is that therapists need to use supervision or consultation with a senior colleague for issues arising in their work which might develop into problems with confidentiality. Such issues might be around crimes committed by patients, information about terrorism or drug-trafficking, the risk of suicide and allegations or suspicions of ongoing child abuse. These situations occur rarely but are likely to be complex when they do emerge. Ethical practice requires therapists to avoid acting hastily on their own and to seek advice sooner rather than later in cases of serious risk, complaint or litigation.

Supervisors may find themselves carrying more responsibility than formerly for containing anxiety and tension, while helping their supervisees to focus on the patient's best interests in increasingly complex situations. If the therapeutic alliance has broken down, the therapist may need the supervisor's support in appealing to his or her employing agency or therapy association. Most complaints can be resolved informally, but more complainants than previously are using professional-conduct procedures. This may be in line with the greater number of people using therapy and their being more aware and discerning. The umbrella organizations, BACP, UKCP and BCP, offer help and advice services and usually have access to lawyers for extra advice. Belatedly, these umbrella organizations have formed an informal joint committee that meets twice a year to share information and ideas on ethical issues.

CONCLUSION

This chapter has outlined some of the difficulties confronting the therapy profession as a result of the movements in our society towards more openness, transparency and accountability, especially regarding keeping personal data and the use that lawyers and others may make of these. Supervisors are likely to find their supervisees increasingly bringing situations from their clinical work of intermeshed process and contextual complications. Involvement with professionals in other disciplines, such as law and medicine, can lead to failures of communication through misunderstanding owing to different meanings attached to the same words or concepts.

Effort is needed to rethink and redefine the confidentiality therapists offer to patients and how this is to be handled. Responsibility cannot be left to patients to inform themselves on their rights and what to expect in therapy. The therapist must ensure that their patients are adequately informed and account for how this responsibility is discharged. The therapy profession, in line with developments in other professions, is in the process of a paradigm shift in the power differential between the 'provider', therapist or supervisor, and the 'user', patient or supervisee. The medical model of paternalistic authority, into whose hands the trusting patient relinquishes responsibility for him- or herself, is no longer the rule. In the medical profession itself, patients are being given and are claiming the right and responsibility to play a part in the course of their treatment. Paternalism is being replaced by a much more equal partnership between two autonomous subjects with different roles but sharing responsibility for the enterprise they embark on together.

Supervisors and their supervisees need to be clear about how recent developments in the law and ethical attitudes affect their responsibilities to their patients, colleagues and profession and adjust their way of working accordingly. Therapists today bear the tensions inherent in working in a highly complex profession that can offer them guidelines for ethical values and principles but no certainties or absolutes. They can find themselves beset by a multitude of situational problems and difficult decisions to be made and, therefore, should equip themselves with a sound contextual, as well as theory, base and seek consultation sooner rather than after a situation has reached crisis point. Reflective practice requires therapists to be aware of when and how their various responsibilities might conflict with each other or with their personal values. Periodic review is important for clarity about policies and contracts, especially with regard to confidentiality and keeping notes and records. Policy should include for what purpose anything is written and for how long it is to be kept. The aim is to develop an ethical attitude through thoughtful reflective practice. Furthermore, the profession needs to develop effective training to produce supervisors skilled in reflecting with their supervisees and supporting them in finding the best option in their patient's interest when difficult and risky decisions loom.

REFERENCES

BACP (2002) Ethical Framework for Good Practice in Counselling and Psychotherapy. Booklet obtainable from BACP: 1 Regent Place, Rugby, CV21 2PJ (email: bacp@bacp.co.uk).

Bingham (2003) Confidentiality: an interdisciplinary issue. British Journal of Psychotherapy 19(4): 467–481.

Data Protection Act (1998) obtainable from: Data Protection Register, Wycliffe House, Water Lane, Wilmslow SK9 5AF.

Dehn C (1995) 'The Woolf Report: against the public interest'. In Zuckerman AAS, Cranston R (eds), Reform and Civil Procedure: Essays on 'Access to Justice'. Oxford: Clarendon Press.

Godley W (2001) 'Saving Masud Khan'. The London Review of Books 23 (4 February): 4–10.

Murdin L (1998) 'The ethical dimensions of supervision'. In Clarkson P (ed.), Supervision: Psychoanalytic and Jungian Perspectives. London: Whurr Publishers.

Thorpe C (2003) Confidentiality: an interdisciplinary issue, introduction to Lord Bingham's address. British Journal of Psychotherapy 19(4): 465–483.

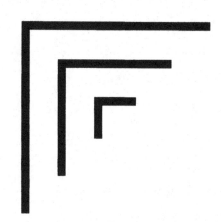

ONTOLOGICAL ASPECTS OF SUPERVISION

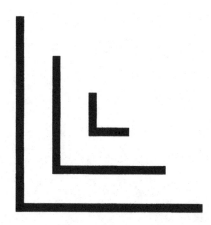

CHAPTER 11
SHAME IN SUPERVISION

EDWARD MARTIN

Man is the only animal that blushes, or needs to.   (Mark Twain 1897)

A MYTH OF THE ORIGINS OF SHAME

At the beginning of the Pentateuch (the first five books of the Old Testament), there are two well-known creation myths. In the first, the Creator operates from a distance, like a grand designer overseeing a miraculous conception. In the second, the Creator is more personally involved with the evolution of the created world, appearing as a craftsman in intimate contact with that which he or she makes. It is in this myth that original man and original woman, aided and abetted by a snake, eat of the tree of the knowledge of good and evil. The immediate result of eating this inviting and luscious fruit appears to be the recognition of separateness and nakedness, the couple covering their genitals and hiding from the Creator. When asked why they are hiding, they admit to an awareness of their nakedness and the source of that knowledge. A heavenly panic sets in, with the Creator voicing fear that having eaten of one tree and gaining consciousness they may find the other somewhat grander tree, that of life and death. If they eat from that, the Creator argued, they would become like us, as Gods, abandon their humanity and become immortal. That must be made impossible (forbidden), and so the die is cast for the human race: they will bear the burden of consciousness, including the knowledge of their own mortality.

About 400 years separate the writing of the final edition of the Genesis myths (900 BC) and the date of the writing of the book of Job. Both concern an amoral Creator whom Jung describes as being 'eaten up with rage and jealousy' and in whom 'insight existed alongside obtuseness, loving-kindness along with cruelty, creative power with destructiveness'. A Creator who appears to need 'conscious man even though, through sheer unconsciousness, he would like to prevent him from being conscious' (Jung 1969: para. 575). Jung suggests that this is 'conceivable only when no reflecting consciousness is present at all, or where the capacity for reflection is very feeble' (Jung 1969: para. 600), a condition suffered at times equally by the Creator and the created.

In the myth of the tree of the knowledge of good and evil, 'lust to the eyes and lovely to look at' (Alter 1996: 12), why are fig leaves chosen, and why hide from the Creator? We might suspect that such an amoral Creator wanted this defiance and might therefore have sought the disguise of a snake to ensure it happened. The knowledge that Adam and Eve gain after eating the fruit is simple: they learn that they are separate. In human development, this represents the point in time when the infant suddenly experiences that the security of the dyadic relationship is not water-tight. Suddenly, the infant's response to a stranger is one of anxiety, 'shyness', manifested in its wanting to hide inside the mother. A painful moment for the child and, if the 'stranger' is father or grandparent, for the adult also. The creation myth can also symbolize a later developmental phase, the moment when the adult (Yahweh in this instance) stumbles uninvited into the children's world catching them out in 'forbidden' play; perhaps as boys and girls engage in mutual genital examination to explore their external differences. Even if sensitively handled, such moments of uncovering may continue to be recalled many years after the event has passed, with an inner if not outward blush.

In the examination of this myth, the offshoots of stranger anxiety are clearly illustrated. It impacts on and affects Oedipal anxiety (Adam and Eve primitively cover themselves); the influence of the superego (God walking in the garden) and the breakdown of narcissistic grandiosity in that Adam and Eve do not go on to eat of the grander tree that would equate them with gods and grant eternal life. The rudimentary nature of their clothes suggests that the human condition is one in which we always remain as naked as the day we were born. In a collective sense, this myth illustrates how separation and anxiety lead to a sense of nakedness, exposure and shame in relation to the objects to which the individual relates. In this case the 'object' is the Creator, but equally it can be the 'gods' of the internal world, our internal objects, the personal, parental and archetypal imagos with which we struggle.

THE PSYCHOLOGICAL GENESIS OF SHAME

The emotion of shame has attracted the attention of a number of writers including Nathanson (1987), Hultberg (1988), Jacoby (1994) and Lidmilla (1997). While shame can be described as a hidden emotion (Hultberg 1988), it has very visible physiological symptoms. Feelings of shame can haunt individuals for years after the shaming event has occurred.

Shame has its genesis early in life but developmentally has many triggers. It is generally conceded that an anticipatory form of shame is stranger anxiety, detectable in infants of around eight to ten months. This is the time when the infant still needs maternal security, to feel at one with the breast/mother, but is on the cusp of recognizing separation. This experience brings with it feelings of vulnerability, anxiety, exposure and loss and the emergence of stranger anxiety, one of the 'shame family of emotions' (Wurmser 1987), which can be defined as a moment of exposure that reveals aspects of the self of a peculiarly sensitive and vulnerable nature.

After this period has been negotiated, others follow fast. For example, failure to master a function, such as bladder or bowel control, within a critical period, usually in a time generally expected by society or by the parents' own agenda, is one of them. The parental response to early manifestation of genital sexuality is another, particularly when the infant has achieved objective self-awarenenss and is in the throes of real genital excitement rather than idle exploration. Rejection or censure to this by an anxious parent is likely to act as a real stimulus to shame. This is thoroughly researched by Nathanson (1987: 39–45), particularly in regard to the development of a 'primary Oedipal complex', which is different from the classical Oedipal complex. The effects of these events on later life have been the subject of much analytic work demonstrating that later experiences of shame may well have their genesis in the early developmental phases of life.

Shame can be experienced when there is a discrepancy between a person's ideals, their introjects and their actual behaviour. Thus the memory of arriving incorrectly dressed for a function can produce at least an internal blush a decade or so later. As the music hall artist put it, 'Fancy going to a funeral in *brown* boots!' Shame can equally be the result of being too fat, too thin, of having the wrong accent, of being a poor scholar or a good all-rounder. Of the two emotions, perhaps it is shame that leaves the deeper scar, that of total abandonment by society, and it is for this reason guilt is sometimes used to defend against shame. Hultberg reminds the readers of Keats' meaningful phrase, 'The most unhappy hours in our lives are those in which we recollect times past to our own blushing – If we are immortal that must be Hell' (Hultberg 1988: 115).

While emotions of shame and guilt are often paired together, clear distinctions need to be made between the two. Guilt is usually associated with offending against ethical and moral principles in thought or action, omission or commission. Feelings of guilt cause feelings of badness. Shame in contrast to guilt is not about ethical or moral principles, the 'should-laws' of philosophical ethics (Jacoby 1994: 1). Guilt is linked to ego, but shame is linked to a total sense of self. It is, as the quotation at the head of this chapter suggests, something genetic, archetypal, to the human race. If its symptoms are spectacularly obvious, the causes frequently remain unconscious. Generally, shame is accompanied by a feeling of nakedness or exposure, a need to be covered. Shame is central in the first few chapters of the Bible, centred around the myth of the Fall, which linked shame to nakedness. The result of Adam's sin, the 'abuse of his liberty', was the 'loss of the grace of conformity to the image of God' (Cross 1957: 994), and so, from the early days of the formation of the Christian Church, the link between concupiscence (desire and lust) and shame was firmly established, and for a time, in popular parlance, the word 'shame' became a euphemism for human genitalia.

In an age where nakedness appears to be no longer a moral problem, confined to an era long past, it is still an age in which the media and the entertainment world know that nakedness will increase their number of viewers or readers. In an age when consciously at least the sin of concupiscence is far from our conscious mind, the warmth of a reddening face still has the ability to trip up the most secular of us and that includes supervisors. Clothed with good training as they are, they can still succumb to some unconscious prompt from within that re-enacts some ancient drama based on an archetypal theme, a parallel process to the conscious communication from the supervisee happening at that moment, and they will feel naked. While shame and/or guilt, the response to committing an ethical offence, may regrettably occur occasionally in supervision, this chapter will be more concerned with aspects of shame that, while they can result in the subject feeling confused and totally worthless, are not connected with any ethical offence having been committed.

EXPOSURE, SHAME AND MUTATIVE INTERPRETATION IN THE THERAPEUTIC SETTING

Within the therapeutic relationship, the 'moment of exposure' and the introduction of 'something strange' occurs when an interpretation is made. Strachey (1934), for instance, notes that therapists experience emotional difficulties when making mutative interpretations, precisely because it entails a moment of exposure. Strachey offers an understanding of the 'constant temptation for the therapist to do something else instead' such as ask questions, or give reassurances or advice. He suggests that 'giving of a mutative interpretation is a crucial act for the analyst as well as for the patient, and that he [the analyst] is exposing himself to some great danger in doing so' (Strachey 1934: 158–159). What is the nature of this danger? Caper (1999) suggests that, having made a mutative interpretation, the therapist often feels retrospectively that its content has been obvious, almost banal, 'often embarrassingly so' – a feeling of nakedness. Accompanying this is the fear that this might spoil the good feeling relationship between therapist and patient, which might lead to the therapist's attempting to promote a superficial and manic warm feeling, 'the maintenance of which depends on the absence of critical thought' (Caper 1999: 39). This suggests a resemblance to Bion's description of a basic assumption mentality, a psychological state that is characterized in groups by similar feelings and avoidances. Caper goes on to suggest that the making of a mutative interpretation requires, amongst other things, that the therapist's ego struggle with the guilt and anxiety produced by his archaic superego. This, 'augmented in its guilt-producing activities by the patient's archaic superego', is opposed to the mutative interpretation. A successful mutative interpretation is therefore 'a victory of ego over superego' (Caper 1999: 44).

How is this threat characterized? Mutative interpretation involves the giving of the therapist (the therapist's breast/penis) to the patient. The patient may respond in a positive, (grateful), admiring, loving, savouring, ingesting way or, in a negative, (ungrateful), ignoring, spoiling, sicking-up manner making it into something persecutory. This happens regardless of how accurate or relevant the interpretation may be. Immediately after a mutative interpretation is made, the therapist will be alert to the patient's response, possibly feeling a personal emptiness and, perhaps, fleetingly, anxiety. The patient may respond immediately, after some silence, or not at all. The therapist may feel a need to say something more, perhaps rationalizing that the interpretation may not have been clear or complete enough. Perhaps this need represents at least in part an attempt to cover up, to put a fig leaf or two in place to cover feelings of nakedness (Nathanson 1987: 4). For even after a long therapeutic relationship has been established, the therapist may suddenly find that in the transference 'mother' has become 'father' and that the patient's response to him may change. The patient may have registered a sudden lack of connection in the transference and the therapist has suddenly become a 'not therapist'. The patient appropriately responds with 'stranger anxiety', that precursor to the feeling of shame.

Shame, unlike guilt, connects the patient or therapist to an internal fantasy audience of internal objects to which the victim feels exposed. It is that sense of nakedness, separation and exposure internally which generates the full affect of shame. This may result in an embarrassing secret being kept hidden for a long time before eventually being shared with the therapist. If disclosure does not occur, the shameful feelings may need to be elucidated upon by reference to the therapist's countertransference and/or reconstruction. As the therapist exposes what the patient feels is shameful, the patient feels understood. The patient might also fantasize that, at the very least, the therapist too has experienced some similar feelings or similar circumstances. The mutative interpretation that links a patient to the therapist both as an object outside him- or herself and at the same time a previously unrecognized internal object exposes both therapist and patient. They are together yet apart and facing something that feels 'naked', 'exposing' and 'shameful', and yet simultaneously this allows for something to be integrated and understood.

SHAME IN SUPERVISION

While the supervisor has a more complex task attempting to understand the multifaceted transference and countertransference between the patient and supervisee, supervisor and supervisee and, through the reflection process, supervisor and patient, similar emotional difficulties are reported to be experienced by supervisors to those experienced by therapists whom Strachey (1934) observed.

Supervision is sometimes described as a lonely task. Paradoxically this seems particularly so in group supervision when, after the supervision has ended, the supervisor leaves the group to their own devices. More than one supervisor has described a fantasy that the group go on to the pub, possibly to talk about the work, or the supervision or the supervisor, while the supervisor in question makes for home alone. Perhaps this feeling of aloneness stems from the supervisor's self-exposure to the group and therefore links to feelings of exposure that are encountered when making a mutative interpretation.

I have suggested earlier (Martin 2002) that supervision should be therapeutic for the supervisee and that this need not detract from the prime supervisory concern, that of caring for the patient. I was not advocating any blurring of boundaries between therapy and supervision: therapeutic supervision requires firmly delineated inner and outer boundaries. My suggestion came as a result of supervising many qualified and capable therapists who had already undergone a long training/personal therapy/analysis. Supervision was being used to keep the unconscious links alive, a weekly or fortnightly workout, similar to a training session for an athlete or musician. During this workout, one will inevitably encounter the shadow, 'the thing a person has no wish to be' (Jung 1966a: para. 470), or, one might add, has no wish to know about. This is clearly demonstrated in the case study below, in which in the shadow of the 'gallant therapist' lay the seducer. Working with the unconscious shadow in supervision therefore carries on the process the supervisee started in their training therapy. The 'less the shadow is embodied in the individual's conscious life, the blacker and denser it is' (Jung 1969: para. 131). Jung's statement suggests that constant familiarity with the shadow is essential for ethical therapy – what better place to (re-)encounter it than in supervision? But bringing the shadow to conscious thought requires exposure and nakedness and the risk of shame.

Yahweh, as portrayed in the myth at the beginning of this chapter, shares with the Yahweh described in the book of Job a need for the fix of applause or worship rather than the rigour of criticism. The good supervisor will, of course, have learnt not to be a Yahweh but recognize that challenge and support are *both* needed to enable the therapist to keep creative. Jung makes the seductive suggestion that women are very suitable as supervisors for male therapists for they 'have excellent intuition . . . trenchant critical insight . . . see what men have up their sleeves . . . see aspects the man does not see' (Jung 1963: 156).

However, his lack of insight was not lost on his former patient Sabina Spielrein (Jung 1963) who, despite being engaged in a deep erotic transference/countertransference relationship with him, was never totally seduced by Jung. In this instance, Jung exemplifies the blindness of the Yahweh of the book of Job as someone who can understand the moral sense of what he is about but at the same time is totally blind to his own amoral behaviour (Jung 1969: para. 573). According to the writer of the book of Job, what unconscious Yahweh has forgotten about and defends himself against obtaining is his need for conscious reflection. Yahweh's need of sycophantic applause caused him to forget that his 'friend and plaything from the beginning of the world' (Jung 1969: para. 617), Sophia, might have something to offer. What Jung is suggesting is that supervision requires wisdom, that which he found embodied in the form of Sophia. 'Who of all that are is a more cunning workman than she?' (Jung 1969: para. 613). Wisdom is not, of course, the prerogative of a supervisor but comes about in making conscious unconscious processes, the shared function of therapy and supervision. Exalted as Sophia may be, her task with Yahweh, like that of supervisor to supervisee, is a lowly one.

In the introduction to her collection of essays concerning that which 'keeps us awake at night, into issues of privacy and publishing, exposure and shame', Jaqueline Rose (Rose 2003: 6/7) cites a poem by Christina Rossetti in which Rose proposes that the poet is saying to the reader 'listen to what I *won't* be telling you' (my italics). Rose then appreciatively suggests that 'psychoanalysis in its best moments still keeps open (the question) – of how on earth to give shape and voice to what one would prefer not to have experienced, (what) one would rather forget' (my parentheses), a task 'not so much to undo forgetting, but to put poetry back into the mind' (Bollas in Rose 2003: 7). In other words, to enable the encountering of the shadow, to think the unthinkable and to transform through the creativity of insight.

So, just when the writer of Job could no longer suffer Yahweh to behave any more like a clueless and thoughtless human being, Wisdom was introduced and with her the chance to allow self-reflection, now an imperative necessity, to happen (Jung 1969: para. 617). And with her introduction, poetry of great beauty:

> I came out of the mouth of the Most High
> and covered the earth like mist
> I had my tent in the heights
> And my throne is a pillar of cloud . . .
> I am like a vine putting out graceful shoots
> My blossoms bear the fruit of glory and wealth . . .
> Approach me, you who desire me
> And take your fill of my fruits.
>
> (*The Jerusalem Bible*, the book of Ecclesiasticus,
> chapter 24 verses 3–7, 17–26)

Likewise, supervision at its best can offer insights to an otherwise blinkered or stuck therapist enabling the words to say it to become the poetry of the transference. Thus the case that follows illustrates aspects of shame that, while they may have their roots in 'stranger anxiety', illustrate Oedipal difficulties encountered in narcissistic defences of a supervisee.

A male therapist, newly qualified, worked for an institution that had developed its own rather superficial training. The organization requested that he work on his own at a subcentre situated in the back room of a town hall. Other than a security guard, he was the only person on site for three hours one evening each week. The focus was on a three-month therapy with a young female patient, his last patient of the day, who presented as having sexual difficulties with her male partner.

At the time of the therapy, the supervisory arrangement was for fortnightly group supervision. In addition, all current cases were discussed at a quarterly individual meeting with a female tutor/supervisor. The therapist had not taken this particular case to the supervision group earlier because there appeared to be no reason to do so.

A feature of the therapeutic relationship, brought to light in the individual review, was that the supervisee consciously thought that he must be sure to behave very correctly towards this patient. Hence, he always allowed a few minutes to elapse between the patient's leaving at the end of the session and his own departure. However, on one particular evening shortly before the review, when the supervisee made to leave the building, he found the patient standing in the doorway of the building, helpless, unprotected, gazing at a torrential rainstorm. The therapist's car was parked immediately outside and he knew his route home passed her house. 'Gallantly' (!) he offered her a lift, dropped her outside her house and went on his way.

He mentioned this in passing to the supervisor/tutor but then found himself feeling embarrassed when she chose to concentrate on this incident. This enabled him to recall a number of issues that, had they been accessible to him previously, might have prompted him to see this case as very suitable to bring to group supervision earlier. For instance, when his patient arrived she usually took off an outer coat or jacket revealing a large expanse of bare back that, even when taking the room size into account, encroached on his personal space. Further, the therapist recognized that he looked forward to her session and realized that he compensated for this by being very 'correct' in his dealings with her. He also recalled that soon after the patient commenced therapy the security guard interrupted a session with a non-urgent message. He was aware that her sexuality had certainly registered with the guard although the supervisee had repressed his response to it. Nothing of the above was ever discussed with the patient in the sessions.

Working in supervision, the therapist was able to admit how attractive this patient was to him. He recognized a mixture of shame feelings – of excitement, of knowing he had sailed close to the wind giving the woman a lift home, and of his unconscious anger directed towards the mother/institution. All these feelings were repressed until they were exposed in supervision. He also realized he would tell himself to be very correct in his outward responses to the patient, thus repressing the unconscious 'seducer', at that point part of his shadow.

Perhaps modelling a creative and symbolic use of nakedness, the tutor/supervisor revealed herself to the therapist both as a senior practitioner and as a woman. This was not a session about technique, about ethics or about therapeutic discipline, although it covered all of these and more. Primarily, it was imparting wisdom (Sophia's domain in Jung's thought) to a neophyte therapist and supervisee. Becoming an effective therapist is not about keeping erotic secrets to yourself but about using them interpretatively in the service of the patient. Secrets tend to become abusive, and in this case the therapist was using a lot of energy in his conflict between feelings of wanting to seduce this attractive needy woman and wanting to keep the therapeutic container safe. Perhaps in the supervision the supervisor/tutor, by revealing her own femininity, her knowledge and her skills, enacted a parallel process showing a back that was not an area of sensual flesh but had a spine in it, doing so in the service of the patient (and future patients) therapeutically, thus moving the supervisee on from responding to the patient as an unconscious category (Eve/seductive woman) (see chapter 1) to a conscious awareness of an identifiable patient with whom he had an asymmetrical relationship. The supervisor's skill enabled the supervisee to expose shame feelings that he defended against sharing in group supervision. It should be added that in this work the supervisor did not self-reveal but worked with the therapist interpretatively within the triangle of supervision. This empathic response enabled the therapist to 'know' the supervisor had 'met him' within herself, thus enabling him to bear feelings of shame without being overwhelmed by them.

SHAME AND EXPOSURE

Psychoanalytic psychotherapy requires that one party reveals personal material to another, who reveals very little of him- or herself in return. Supervision, on the other hand, is a more open dialogue in which supervisors may be more self-revealing than they would be when working as therapists. Supervision therefore can become an arena where, as the novelist Pat Barker puts it, the past 'continues to haunt, influence, distort and occasionally redeem the present' (Jaggi 2003: 16). What is kept in, allowed out, taken in, given out, forms the matrix of emotional life. Psychotherapists *before* their training have introjected society's values and norms that *during* the training are subjected to modification. While the result of offending against professional ethics should result in a blush of shame, paradoxically, a similar blush may be the result of offending against the introjected system of values in pursuit of the therapeutic endeavour.

Supervision is the arena in which it is possible (desirable?) to share the *excitement* of the psychoanalytic work with another. Stoller refers to excitement as a 'dialectic, a rapid oscillation between two possibilities (and their affects). One we tell ourselves has a positive, the other a negative outcome: pleasure/pain, relief/trauma, success/failure, danger/safety. Between the two lies risk. The synthesis is the creative product: daydream, pornography, painting, symphony, religious ritual, drama' (Stoller 1979: 7) and, dare one add, supervision? While excitement in supervision may be generated by the parallel process involving the absent patient, it can also be generated between supervisor and supervisee alone. Excitement or zeal (enthusiastic ardour) may allow one or other of the participants to let something slip out ('by mistake') resulting in feelings of shame. That which is private and 'nobody's business' becomes unintentionally quite visible and exposed. This can be followed by 'the shameful brooding over what one has "given away" of oneself in an uncontrolled way, or by doubts about what one has "left behind"' (Jacoby 1994: 52).

To be *found empty* or to have nothing to give or suggest is a dread that haunts many a new supervisor. The feeling of shame for not coming up to the mark, of knowing that someone less experienced than you is stronger, more insightful or more skilled than you, can easily resonate with earlier feelings of competitiveness and inadequacy. However, feeling empty could also be a countertransference response to the supervisee's feelings of shame of having to go to supervision. The supervisee might be unconsciously attempting to attack the supervisor. This need to diminish the supervisor might be shown through the supervisee's asking for an obscure book reference or testing out some newly acquired piece of theory to see if the supervisor is up to scratch: shaming by projection, as it were.

The use of supervisory knowledge, as opposed to *supervisory wisdom*, may also result in feelings of shame for the supervisor. To display cleverness may feel more like performing than enabling, and the shameful fear might be that the supervision session had been used to satisfy the supervisor's narcissism rather than the needs of the supervisee/patient. On the other hand, wisdom, with its overtones of sagacity, discretion, insight and tact, suggests more of a drawing out of the supervisee. The supervisor can then feel protected, enabling the supervisee to use their own knowledge and create their own wisdom.

SHAME AND FORGIVENESS

In a shame society the committing of an offence is punished by exclusion. Historically, offenders were executed outside the walls of the city. The recent London transport company's publicity campaign to prevent fare avoidance chose a shame motif. 'What colour would you choose when caught without your ticket?' ask prominently placed placards showing the choice of a range of reds. The suggestion is that when caught avoiding paying one's fare the offender would be shamed, visibly physiologically marked and feel excluded from and outside of the community of the remaining passengers.

The case study described earlier in this chapter was used with a number of training groups for trainee supervisors. The facilitators were surprised and at times shocked that a number of trainees would have chosen shame tactics to deal with the supervisee had they been the supervisor. They would for instance have exposed him to his professional body, with the accompanying fantasy that that would result in disciplinary measures being adopted, his name being published as an offender and that he would be excluded from the therapeutic community. In some cases, the vehemence was such that it felt as though he should be hung up to dry outside the therapeutic community's walls. Such I think is the power of shame and the responsibility of supervisors to be aware that in supervision long-repressed aspects of the shadow can manifest themselves in both supervisees and supervisors.

In contrast, in a guilt society, the offender is punished within and, technically, once the punishment has been served, the offender is reunited with society. He or she may be formally forgiven, ritually by a priest or personally by his or her victim. He or she may, however, still feel shame, and shame can be very personal and lasting. Perhaps feelings of shame have to be more resolved than forgiven, a movement, in Kleinian (Hinshlewood 1989: 373) terminology, from the paranoid-schizoid to the depressive position.

In this connection, it would be incomplete if the paranoid/persecutory thoughts the supervisee in the case study experienced were not mentioned. He did not (as some feared) get away 'scot free'! Through therapy, he was able to embrace aspects of the shadow and feel his erotic feelings and sexuality to be less dangerous and could be used more creatively. He was also able to allow an experience of the supervisor not as an all-seeing persecutory god but as symbolic of wisdom. In other words, he was able to give up sufficient of his narcissistic grandiosity and persecutory anxiety in relation to 'right or wrong' to experience the 'depressive position'. Thus, the supervisee in the case study was eventually able to resolve his feelings about his early mistake. Over years, the tendency to blush at the memory faded. However such an outcome is not universal, and it is not uncommon that many years after a shaming event it is still possible to trigger a resurgence of the apparently forgotten blushing shame.

SHAME AND THE SUPERVISION OF SUPERVISION

Mattinson's (1981) seminal paper *The Deadly Equal Triangle* focuses on the supervision of supervision. During a workshop, participants were invited to bring their supervision work for discussion. While running the workshop, Mattinson discovered a puzzling phenomenon. Although the participants had voluntarily chosen to join the workshop and had consciously agreed to the task of presenting sessions for discussion, great difficulty arose in persuading them to actually present this work. The accuracy of Mattinson's observations of this workshop will have been verified by many who have participated in the supervision of supervision. There has often been a reluctance to discuss work, and even when this reluctance is overcome it seems easier to talk *about* a session than details of *the interaction*, especially the supervisor's actual comments and the supervisee's responses to them. Mattinson suggests that the clue to this difficulty lay in the Oedipal nature of the relationship with the intrusion of a third into a dyad. This is familiar territory. Such intrusions will have been experienced universally from the early months of life; therefore, the intrusion of the third in supervision will unconsciously be linked to the 'shame family of emotions'.

If care is not taken with the boundaries, the supervision of supervision can provide a temptation to play around, even play with fire, by avoiding the task. Here the professional seniors may be tempted to play as gods. They may then run the risk of being like human Semele, who instead of recognizing her limitations insisted on having intercourse with the god Zeus unclothed (without his human disguise) and was burnt to death as a result. For in this arena it is possibly more difficult to admit one's inadequacies and appear nakedly human. The danger and risk is of projecting onto colleagues the stature of a God taking a supervisory stroll in his kingdom rather than attempt to become 'nakedly' human within the supervisory task.

While Mattinson does not actually refer directly to 'shame' in her paper, its presence abounds. Examples given are those of the too quickly promoted supervisor who is insecure about what he or she can offer to supervisees, the concern of supervisors feeling they are 'senior' and therefore should be expected to 'know' (be clothed as it were) and the tendency for supervisors to suggest their supervisees close cases when the length of therapy has exceeded the supervisor's own therapeutic experience. In all these three examples, supervisors are placed in the position of eating of the tree of knowledge and, having done so, feel naked and therefore attempt to find a hiding place. Oedipal in nature as the supervision of supervision is, shame would appear to be a prominent emotion. A peer group can particularly amplify such feelings because the dynamics of the peer group, like the gang, include sibling rivalry. Can the presenter risk the exposure of admitting to not knowing or to have broken the group rules, or speaking the group language? Can he or she repeat the shame of feeling a misfit but not knowing why, the shame of feeling a failure in competition with shortcomings in knowledge of theory or in clinical skill? (Wurmser 1987; Nathanson 1987: 4).

CONCLUSION

Mythologically, the experience of shame leads to individuation. Adam and Eve are forced out of a dyadic relationship in the garden womb to 'till their own soil' or, in other words, 'to divest their selves of false wrappings of the persona and of the suggestive power of primordial images' (Jung 1966b: 269). Experiences of shame, with their root in 'stranger anxiety', embrace unresolved aspects of supervisee/patient psyches that include narcissistic defence organization and an overdominant archaic superego (and thus an underdeveloped beneficent superego). The supervisor needs to embrace an understanding of these aspects of their psyche by self-exploration to enable supervisees to recognize these aspects in themselves and their absent patients to ensure the elusive goal of integration and individuation is not blocked.

REFERENCES

Alter R (1996) Genesis. New York and London: W Norton and Company.

Caper R (1999) 'On the difficulty of making a mutative interpretation'. In A Mind of One's Own. London: Routledge.

Cross FL (ed.) (1957) The Oxford Dictionary of the Christian Church. London: Oxford University Press.

Hinshlewood RD (1989) A Dictionary of Kleinian Thought. London: Free Association Books.

Hultberg P (1988) Shame – a hidden emotion. Journal of Analytical Psychology 33(2): 109–126.

Jacoby M (1994) Shame and the Origins of Self-esteem. London: Routledge.

Jaggi M (2003) 'Dispatches from the Front'. In Guardian Review, 16 August.

Jung CG (1963) Memories, Dreams, Reflections. London: Collins.

Jung CG (1966a) The Practice of Psychotherapy. Collected Works 16. London: Routledge.

Jung CG (1966b) Two Essays on Analytical Psychology. Collected Works 7. London: Routledge.

Jung CG (1969) Answer to Job. Collected Works 11. London: Routledge.

Lidmilla A (1997) 'Shame, knowledge and modes of enquiry in supervision'. In Shipton G (ed.), Supervision of Psychotherapy and Counselling: Making a Place to Think. Buckingham and Philadelphia: Open University Press.

Martin E (2002) 'Accessing the absent patient'. In Driver C, Martin E (eds), Supervising Psychotherapy. London: Sage Publications.

Mattinson J (1981) The Deadly Equal Triangle. Northampton, MA, and London: The Smith College School of Social Work and the Group for the Advancement of Psychotherapy in Social Work.

Nathanson DL (ed.) (1987) The Many Faces of Shame. New York and London: Guilford Press.

Rose J (2003) 'Freud in the Tropics'. In On Not Being Able to Sleep. London: Chatto and Windus.

Stoller R (1979) Sexual Excitement. London: Maresfield Library.

Strachey J (1934) The nature of the therapeutic action of psycho-analysis. International Journal of Psycho-Analysis 15(1): 127–159.

Twain M (1897) Following the Equator. Hartford, CT: The American Publishing Company.

Wurmser L (1987) 'The mask of shame'. In Nathanson D (ed.), The Many Faces of Shame. New York and London: Guilford Press.

CHAPTER 12

SUPERVISION AS SELF-QUESTIONING

THE CONTRIBUTION OF JUNG'S *PSYCHOLOGICAL TYPES* TOWARDS THEORY IN SUPERVISION

MICHAEL WHAN

> *Every theory we hold practices upon us in one way or another, so that ideas are always in practice and do not need to be put there.* (James Hillman 1992: 123)

INTRODUCTION

Jung's book *Psychological Types* (1976) deals not so much with 'personality types', that is whether a person's basic *attitude* is introverted or extraverted, whether a person's *function* is feeling, thinking, intuition, or sensation, or these in various combination. Rather, it is concerned with the interior life of psychology as a discipline, *with the soul of psychology itself.* Jung seeks to show how these fundamental attitudes and ways of apprehending and comprehending oneself and the world operate in the very making of psychology, as well as in religious, aesthetic, ethical and philosophical notions of all kinds. Jung suggests that a psychological theory may orient itself in its basic attitude as essentially 'introverted' or 'extraverted', as governed more by, say, 'thinking' or 'feeling' or 'intuition', and so on.

Further, behind such personal traits of one's typology, he detected a certain archetypal or impersonal inflection, the 'numinal accent' (Jung 1976: para. 982), which a priori falls selectively on one or other attitude and function. Hillman considers that the term 'numinal' indicates something 'divine . . . the structuring power of a type is like that of an archetype or mythologem', which suggests that typological theory is more complex than the straightforward empirical description of 'personality types' (Hillman 1980: 21).

In recalling Freud's sexual libido theory, Jung asserts that 'for Freud, sexuality was undoubtedly a *numinosum*', concluding, 'Freud . . . must himself be profoundly affected by the power of Eros that he actually wished to elevate it into a dogma . . . like a religious numen' (Jung 1963: 152–154). Thus, Jung locates an archetypal factor at work in Freud's theorizing – a veritable *daimon* (a tutelary, attendant spirit; the personification of an inner guiding voice; that which allots one's fate). In thinking about psyche, Freud was seized by an 'idea' which was itself archetypal – that is a universal symbolic image, value and dynamic inflected through the subjective complexes of Freud's personality, namely Freud's 'personal equation' (James 1961). Thus *all* psychological theory reflects the personality and typology of its 'creator', and, in addition, personality and typology are themselves deeply influenced by the archetypal background of the psyche.

Supervision, as an attempt to reflect *psychologically* on the psychological work of analysis, psychotherapy and counselling, works within this overlap of the personal and archetypal. It finds itself ever in the midst of the psyche and its *logos*, psychology and its bearings have to be taken from *within the field* in which it is always and already deeply immersed. Psychological theories and concepts need themselves to be regarded as living forms, expressions, of a kind of deeper subjectivity or agency, which (as with Freud's theory of sexuality, Eros) possess us and formatively shape our psychological notions. It is to this question of just how *differently* the various psychologies can understand psyche, say, as between Freud, Jung and Adler, that Jung addresses his work *Psychological Types*.

Jung understood the four functions of his typology, that is feeling, thinking, intuition and sensation, not as a 'map' but rather 'like the four points of the compass' (Jung 1976: para. 958). A historian of psychology, Shamdasani, has closely examined the role of this particular text in relation to Jung's psychological project and raised an underlying question not only in relation to Jung but also with regard to the whole discourse of psychology, namely *whether psychology was and is possible* (Shamdasani 2003). For, if the personal equation is always operative, *can a universal or general psychology be developed at all?* The notion of a psychological typology at work in all psychological theorizing means that problematic factors are at work that all claims for a universalist psychology have to confront. Shamdasani argues that psychology – and hence the analytic psychotherapies dependent upon it – has and have failed to overcome this *aporia* of the *subjectivity of psychological theorizing* (Shamdasani 2003).

In the 'Foreword' to his work, Jung specifically cautions how *not* to read *Psychological Types*. To use it as a 'grid' or 'map' for 'typing' different kinds of personality is to misread Jung's intention, but despite Jung's warning that is precisely the way it has been read and largely put to use, that is essentially as a positivistic application and 'testing' (such as the Grey–Wheelwright and Myers–Briggs typological profiles) in order to determine a person's basic attitudinal type (introversion/extraversion) and one's dominant function(s) of feeling, thinking, intuition or sensation, or some sort of combination of these. Though the Grey–Wheelwright and Myers–Briggs tests were developed to make Jung's typology usable and accessible, this can lead to a misunderstanding of the essential issues Jung is considering.

Another way of employing the typology is clinically, as with the transference and countertransference dynamic (Groesbeck 1978; Bradway and Henderson 1978; Fordham 1972). Useful as this may be as a way into the actual supervisory situation for reflecting on the non-pathological differences between the patient and the supervisee, it still does not adequately take up Jung's challenge. Rather, *Psychological Types* requires a dialectical, psychological, engagement with the underlying theory.

I want to elucidate the contribution of *Psychological Types* to the reflective aspect of the supervisory process, by drawing upon a statement of Jung's: 'Every psychotherapist not only has his own method – he himself is that method' (Jung 1954: 198). Though each psychotherapist *embodies* their 'method' in the thoughts, feelings, fantasies, dreams, utterances, silences and actions of their being, that method cannot be reduced back to them only in a personalistic sense, that is to say it is more than a product derived from their own personal subjectivity. The 'method' receives its warrant from the discourse of psychology itself. Psychology has arisen out of an archetypal and historical (impersonal or transpersonal) background, and the therapist lays claim to working *psychologically* as well as in his or her own singular way.

Psychology unfolds its dialectical life through the singularity of lived moments of the analytic/psychotherapeutic setting. Jung puts it this way: the patient and psychotherapist 'form . . . a coming together . . . and at the same time are symptoms of a certain process or run of events' (Jung 1977a: 421; Giegerich 1998). But of what then is the psychotherapeutic relationship a 'symptom'? The 'coming together' of patient and psychotherapist is itself symptomatic of psychotherapeutic and analytic psychology. Parts of this 'run of events', the transference and countertransference, are not, *in the first place*, brought *to* the analytic setting by the psychotherapist and patient, rather, they are *already solicited by the analytic setting itself* (Holt 1998). This 'run of events' is implicit or inherent in it.

Another way to put this is to conceive of the analytic setting as a dramatic field, *enacted* by the psychotherapist and patient. This calls upon the supervisory process to question the very psychology underlying the psychotherapeutic process. It has to ask questions about the theoretical perspective informing the process, a questioning which goes beyond the psychodynamics of the personal subjectivity of the patient and therapist. It has to reflect upon the 'inner drama' that depth psychology itself is enacting, to glimpse its archetypal background, its dominant images. Such a call throws into question the very way that psychologies, for example psychoanalysis, analytical psychology, psychosynthesis, seek to defend themselves against the dialectic of the soul's self-movement, which manifests as a deep self-questioning.

For it is psychology that mediates and constellates what happens and how it is interpreted in the therapeutic setting, and which inducts both psychotherapist and patient into the therapeutic process: 'Psychological induction inevitably causes the two parties to get involved in the transformation of the third and to be themselves transformed in the process' (Jung 1954: para. 399), and so, whether working as psychotherapists or supervisors, we are drawn unconsciously, induced, as it were, into the psychodynamics of the therapeutic setting. In supervision, this manifests itself as a 'parallel process': something is enacted that causes the pair to reflect on, and seek to understand, what is happening, the constellation of 'the third', and, as supervisors, may become transformed by what is engaged with in supervision.

Supervision's task contributes to the recognition and understanding of this process of induction (transference, countertransference, suggestion, projection, identification, projective identification, hypnotic induction etc.) and to the transformation of the third. And to question this process of induction means that psychology itself cannot be exempted from critical self-reflection, otherwise this may cause a deception which leaves out one of the 'powers that be' operative in the inductive dynamic. Supervisors cannot remain like naive, innocent, unquestioning children in relation to psychological theory and practice, even if that openness to questioning psychotherapy, analysis and psychology themselves makes life very difficult in the world of analytic supervision. It demands of the supervisor a capacity, indeed, a 'negative capability', to remain in an ironic, or even more strongly, *paradoxical* position with regard to the psychological theory or theories he or she works with. It implies a struggling with psychology itself all the time and that it cannot, fundamentally, be taken for granted.

The 'third' that needs to be 'transformed' is psyche itself, the autonomous factor that realizes itself as psychological theory or thinking that is psychology as psyche's consciousness of itself, its self-recognition as psyche. Jung understood the therapeutic process not as a two-person dialogue but rather as a dialectic involving 'three persons'. In his intricate elaboration of this thesis, Giegerich states:

> What is this factor, who is the third person of psychotherapy? It is, of course, the soul, which is no longer imagined as the individual property of each of the two other persons, but must be given independent reality. It is the world of complexes and archetypal images, of views and styles of consciousness, and thus it is also psychology itself . . . including all our ideas about the soul, its pathology and therapy, as well as our Weltanschauung.
> (Giegerich 1977: 153; also see Holt 1987)

This 'third party in the alliance' (Jung 1954: para. 348), itself the psychotherapeutic process, differentiates into 'two aspects or counterparts', namely, 'the soul

itself and the theory about it (psychology)' (Giegerich 1977: 153). For Jung, theory serves not as a dry abstraction but as a living, guiding, shaping spirit in the
analytic encounter. As Giegerich puts it, if 'psychology is in this sense the third
autonomous person with a living and decisive presence in psychotherapy, it
may also be suspected of having its own unconsciousness – and possibly even
its own neurosis' (Giegerich 1977: 153). In this way, supervision has to deal with
three 'patients': the actual patient, the psychopathology of the psychotherapist,
and *psychology itself as patient.* Thus supervision has to engage with this 'third
person', whose presence triangulates, and therefore constellates, both the possibility of the psychopathology of the psychotherapeutic process and its healing
power. For the shaping spirit of psychological theory is triangulating, dialectical. It is both a remedy and a poison. For instance, the supervisory task may
need us to question the very powerfully obsessive way that the 'parent/child'
notion has seized hold of psychotherapeutic psychology, so that we can open
our understanding of the transference and countertransference dynamic to
other factors operating in the psyche. It is not only the patient who may be
obsessed with his or her parent; analytic psychology too is hooked by a 'parental
complex' and needs to see through its own 'guiding fictions'.

According to Hillman, a defensive, pathological aspect within Jung's theory
shows itself, for instance, in the connection between his typology and notion
of the mandala (in Buddhism a 'mandala' is taken as symbolizing the universe
and is seen as an enclosing circle; in Jungian psychology, it represents the
wholeness of the self). Hillman (1980) links both these components of Jung's
theory in terms of Jung's own period of psychological crisis. The timing of
their appearance belongs to that moment in his life which Jung (1963) speaks
of as his 'confrontation with the unconscious' (1913-1919). Typology and mandala, Hillman points out, are in the service of 'ordering irreconcilable conflicts'.
But, he continues:

> Functionally, the interlocking system of the typology and its power of explaining one's
> differences within oneself and the world, as well as one's differences with the world . . .
> serves, as any good system, as an apotropaic or paranoid buttress of ego-consciousness (to
> which Jung attributes the types) against what he called Dionysian dissolution . . .
> We still turn to typology when we need system . . . Our moves in psychology recapitulate
> Jung's moves. Ideas have roots in the necessities of our abnormal psychologies in Jung's
> no less than ours.   (Hillman 1980: 19–20)

In the same way that a mandala can serve defensively against disintegration,
a kind of symbolic protective circle, the symmetrical 'fourfold' typology, Hillman is suggesting, acts against 'Dionysian dissolution' (which refers to varying
states, including a dimming or lowering of consciousness; disintegration anxiety; falling into an ecstatic, altered state of consciousness or being). The genesis

of Jung's typology was, in part, an attempt to account psychologically for the very different theories of Freud and Adler, which, he argued, arose from different attitudinal types, extraversion and introversion respectively, rooted in their personalities. And not least, as he observes, he wrote it as 'a critique of my own psychological peculiarity' (Jung 1976: xi). Yet, notwithstanding Jung's own statement of purpose of *Psychological Types*, Hillman detects the paranoid 'necessity' of an 'abnormal psychology' inherent in the very *systematizing*, 'fourfold', mandalic, activity of (Jung's) psychological typology: psychology, analysis, themselves as an intellectual ego-defence, or what psychoanalysis speaks of as 'the mind object' (Phillips 1995).

What Jung is effectively doing is to throw the whole project of psychology into question. Depth psychology cannot escape the nature of its being and becoming *as a question*, which it becomes when we perceive it as a 'third person' in the psychotherapeutic or supervisory process, and which means that psychology's movement expresses itself through the fluidity of its thought as critical self-reflection, as self-questioning, as dialogue and dialectic. Always *questionable*, psychology is always 'in the making', *always a difficulty to itself*. It cannot escape its inherent difficulty, since every psychology reflects the subjectivity of its creator's personality. To be psychological, to follow its dialectic faithfully, we are always having to make and unmake psychological theory and practice. Whenever any psychology purports to generalize or universalize, it has yet to account for the 'self-overcoming' of its 'personal equation', for its particularity. It has to offer, in Jung's own words, a 'critique' of its 'own psychological peculiarity'.

In his Tavistock Lectures (Jung 1977b) between the two World Wars, Jung opened his discussion by proposing that psychology stood in the way of itself. It was, as it were, at cross-purposes with itself, a limitation that at the same time marked its essential characteristic. Thus, depth psychology becomes *psychological* about itself when it realizes its self-contradictory or dialectical nature. The practitioner of psychology has no choice but to follow psychology's winding path to its innermost, where it folds back on itself. Jung begins by doubting whether the enormity of such an undertaking, namely 'the perplexing and distressingly complicated nature of its subject-matter, the psyche itself' (Jung 1977b: para. 6) can be fully understood. For the psyche is both the object of study of psychology, and its subject. In the personal equation of the psychologist's personality lies a deeper subjectivity, the psyche or soul itself. Hence, the practising psychotherapist has yet, in Jung's estimation of how unconscious we are of the meaning or nature of psychology, to realize the 'menace of so formidably vicious a circle' (Jung 1977b: para. 6). According to Jung, there is no Archimedean or meta-psychological or methodological vantage point from outside the psyche by which one could wholly and objectively make psychological statements. The psyche is ever upon us: 'We should never forget that in any psychological discussion we are not saying anything *about* the psyche, but that the psyche is always speaking about *itself* (Jung 1962: para. 483). Jung elaborates on this 'vicious' or, put otherwise, 'hermeneutic' circle: 'As "pure" psychology its principle of explanation is *ignotum per ignotius* ('naming the unknown by the more unknown'), for it can reconstruct the observed process only in the same medium from which that process is itself constituted' (Jung 1964: para. 162). Thus, *psychological theory and practice are no less subjective expressions of the psyche.*

As such, this dialectical understanding of psychology – that is as both 'subject' and 'object' – carries fundamental implications for the supervisory process. Since supervision seeks to address what is happening in the psychotherapeutic setting itself, implying a certain advantage of understanding, a certain possibility of the greater awareness of the meaning of what is occurring, then it must also admit its own 'subjectivity'. That it too is *subjected to* the effects of psyche. As noted earlier, this means not only the psychodynamics of what is happening in the supervision itself – such as 'parallel process', transference and countertransference, projective identification and so on – but that it also requires an awareness of the effect of psyche in the very theorizing itself. For, as Jung puts it, every 'psychic process, so far as it can be observed as such, is essentially a presentation; and its reconstruction – or "re-presentation" – is at best only a variant of the same presentation' (Jung 1964: para. 162). Our transferences, countertransferences and other psychic factors, such as idealization, denigration and identification, feature not only in relation to supervisor, patient, analyst or psychotherapist but also in relation to theory itself. And theory expresses not only the subjective factor, the 'personal equation', of whoever has thought it into being, whether, say, Klein, Freud, Adler, Jung, Winnicott etc. reflecting their particular complexes and psychic inflections, but also the archetypal level of the psyche.

Theorizing can therefore be seen as both an expression of subjective factors deriving from the individual creator, including the historical forces which have affected him or her, and also of certain archetypal motifs, certain 'root metaphors' that shape culture, language and thought. Such archetypal 'root metaphors' are at work not only in the patient's psyche but also in the supervisory process itself. If we go below the level of abstraction and conceptualization, which usually comprise much theoretical utterance, we come upon a fantasy level. The French psychoanalyst Roustang, writing on the connection between fantasy and theory, observes: 'In order to question analysis, one must first stop being fascinated by theory and analyse the fantasies or desires that gave rise to it; one must analyse theory as the text of a dream or myth' (Roustang 1958: 58). Such analysis requires both supervisor and supervisee to be *psychological* in their approach to psychology itself, not to be naive or remain innocent, to know its history, not only the biographical, but the larger historical context within which it emerged and which shaped it. If not, then, as Roustang says, theory 'becomes the starting point for thinking in general and thus a system in which one is caught. Theory becomes a symptom or a system of defence' (Roustang 1958: 58). We become 'entranced' by theory, by the power of its language, fascinated and forget that it arose as an abstract expression of subjective factors. This is exactly the point that Jung made when he pointed out how Freud had been seized by the notion of 'Eros', and Adler by that of 'power'. Roustang's observation directs us to see through the abstraction of theory to its underlying fantasy base. In Jung's theory, there will be found Jung's fantasies, and, in Freud's theory, Freud's fantasies, and so on.

Jung comprehended the underlying epistemologies of the different psychological theories as themselves reflecting different psychologies, inflected through the personality of the founding psychologist. Generally, he argued, there was a failure to recognize the nature of psychology as both subject and object, and he explicitly understood his own psychology as a subjective 'confession' of his own 'psychological peculiarity'. Supervision then not only is the application of a theory to a particular psychotherapeutic relationship but also holds out the possibility of psychology reflecting upon itself – *supervision as a moment in psychology's inner dialectic with itself*. In supervision what is sought is *absolute subjectivity, absolute interiority* and the task of supervision is to apprehend and comprehend *psychic reality*. Supervision not only looks at the patient's psychic reality but also has to bear in mind that theories too are abstractly formed fantasies or transformed fantasies and desires. We not only have to interpret by way of one or other psychological theory; we also have to see through the theory to its (hidden) subjectivity. In supervision, then, we have to carry the contradictory tension of the psychology we work with as both subject and object.

To regard the theory itself as the absolute truth, however, is to confuse the relative level of subjectivity with the fundamental nature of the psyche as absolute interiority. Hence, the supervisory process gets caught in dogmatic claims, losing touch with the notion of a crucial difference, confusing the relative (the particular theory and mode of practice) with the absolute (the psyche itself). Jung's application of a typology to the making of each psychological theory can be understood as his attempt to maintain this necessary difference, in which the tension between the absolute (the psyche itself) and anything we say about it, or rather, its way of speaking through us, the relative, is maintained. Whenever we speak psychologically of the psyche (absolute interiority), whatever is said comes refracted through the prism of the particular personality of the one claiming to speak psychologically. The failure to recognize both modalities of experience as present in every psychology, that in psychology the psyche is both subject and object, leads on to dogmatic claims. For dogmatism in whatever form arises from the collapse of the difference between the relative and the absolute. Essentially, the dogmatic claim obscures every theory's subjectivity behind a so-called objectivity, thereby losing fundamental differences and constitutive tensions, differences necessary for any deeper psychological reflection. To hold onto this difference, the supervisory process needs to be able to hold itself in the tensions of irony and paradox, which means recognizing the deep levels of subjectivity within the psychological theory and practice it brings to bear. Without such irony and paradox, the supervisory process may become a process of indoctrination, in which questioning of the theoretical frame is prohibited, the typological slant of its 'author' denied, as if she or he saw existence through the privileged eye of the absolute.

This critical difference, 'critical' in the sense that it allows psychological reflection upon psychology itself, is precisely what Jung seeks to clarify and differentiate in *Psychological Types*. It was an aspect of his working on 'the transformation of the third'. Yet this work is often misunderstood, as Jung himself observes in the foreword:

> Far too many readers have succumbed to the error of thinking that Chapter X ('General Description of the Types') represents the essential content and purpose of the book, in the sense that it provides a system of classification and a practical guide to a good judgement of human character . . . This regrettable misunderstanding completely ignores the fact that this kind of classification is nothing but a childish parlour game . . . My typology is far rather a critical apparatus . . . but not in any sense to stick labels on people at first sight. It is not a physiognomy and not an anthropological system, but a critical psychology . . . For this reason I have placed the general typology . . . at the end of the book . . . I would therefore recommend the reader who really wants to understand my book to immerse himself first of all in chapters II and V. He will gain more from them than from any typological terminology superficially picked up, since this serves no other purpose than a totally useless desire to stick on labels.   (Jung 1976: xiv–xv)

At the end of the book, Jung again reiterates the intention of his work: 'Its purpose is rather to provide a critical psychology . . . an attempt . . . to provide an explanatory basis and theoretical framework for the boundless diversity . . . in the formation of psychological concepts' (Jung 1976: paras 986–987). The two key elements here are, first, that Jung intends *Psychological Types* as a 'critical psychology' and, second, as Hillman notes, Jung is less concerned with so-called personality types than with the 'boundless diversity' of 'psychological concepts' (Hillman 1980: 24). Jung's 'critical psychology' draws on typology not as a critique of personality – whether it be Freud's, Adler's or whomever's – rather it is a critical reflection on psychology itself, a kind of epistemological therapy.

To realize just how far Jung's book is from the kind of approach to typology as found in the so-called classification of 'personality types', one has only to follow Jung's own prescription for reading it, recommending the reader to go first to chapters II and V. Chapter II is a profound meditation on the philosophical writings of Friedrich Schiller, particularly *On the Aesthetic Education of Man*, and includes a comparison with Goethe's thought and excursus into Indian metaphysics. Chapter V concerns the problem of typology in poetry, examining Carl

Spitteler's *Prometheus and Epimetheus*, and taking in the connection between the 'worship of the soul' and the 'worship of woman', referring to Dante, and an early Christian text, *The Shepherd of Hermas*, Meister Eckhart, and Grail and vessel symbolism, hardly the stuff of the Grey–Wheelwright and Briggs–Myers tests. Another chapter, VII, focuses on the question of typology in aesthetics, in which Jung offers a subtle discussion of abstraction and empathy in terms of introversion and extraversion.

One of the tasks of supervision consists of mediating the particular work at hand and the theoretical dimension – respectively, the role of empathy and of abstraction. Jung's *Psychological Types* enables a deeper understanding of these two elements of the psychotherapeutic relationship, empathy and abstraction, reflecting on how each represents a fundamentally different way of 'being in the world'. If empathy allows us to enter more fully into another's experiences, abstraction, as the word itself connotes, draws us out of the 'concrete truth' of the particular experience towards theorizing, such is a change in our way of relating, in our 'way of being', towards the recounted events, experiences and feelings reflected on and spoken of in the supervisory encounter. The psychology of abstraction and its role in the constitution of psychological theorizing is different from the role and nature of empathy in psychological thinking and practice. As Jung conceives them, one arises out of a basic anxiety in relation to the introverted relationship to the world; the other derives from an anxiety in relation to the extraverted attitude. Jung understood the function of empathy as the projection of subjective contents. This projection was itself preceded by an opposite unconscious devaluation or depotentiation of the object; the act of devaluation or depotentiation expresses an unconscious fantasy. Thus the 'object is emptied, so to speak, robbed of its spontaneous activity, and thus made a suitable receptacle for subjective contents' (Jung 1976: para. 491). Connecting empathy with the extraverted attitude, Jung is proposing that it has its roots in an unconscious anxiety related to otherness. The act of abstracting is likewise derived from a fundamental anxiety associated with the introverted attitude or approach. For abstraction arises as a response of withdrawal from 'a frighteningly animated world that seeks to overpower and smother' the introverted mind. Abstraction, in Jung's view, serves as 'a saving formula calculated to enhance' one's 'subjective value at least to the point' where one can hold one's 'own against the influence of the object' (Jung 1976: para. 492). Again, this requires of the supervisory task a reflection upon the role of deep psychic fantasies and emotional states of mind in the actual genesis of psychotherapeutic practice and thought. To apply theory, for all that it can offer, may also, at the same time, be a defensive move, speaking a 'language of distance', and arising out of an anxiety constellated in the supervisory situation in response to the psychic material presented. In supervision, then, the very elements of understanding that are brought to bear on case material, empathy and abstraction, may themselves express underlying unconscious fantasies in relation to deep anxieties and defences which underlie the fundamental dispositions with which we approach ourselves, others and the world.

Psychological Types recalls to supervision's reflective process the question of psychology to itself, to which, as a moment in psychology's self-questioning, it is answerable. It directs us to the underlying, unconscious processes that constitute psychological theories. In a 1925 seminar, Jung put this succinctly:

> *With all of this I give you the impure thoughts that lay back of the Types, where I have carried over into abstract terms the contest between the superior and inferior functions, first seen by me in the symbolic form of the slaying of the hero. Such things as I have described in these fantasies speak in symbolic form of things later to become conscious and to take form as abstract thoughts, when they will look altogether different from their plastic origins.*   (Jung 1990: 48–49)

In this brief and seminal statement, Jung exposes not only the fantasy origins of his own psychological theorizing, not only his own 'personal equation', but also the underlying archetypal images at the back of all our 'personal equations', and the constitutive role of both in the genesis of depth and psychotherapeutic psychology.

REFERENCES

Bradway K, Henderson J (1978) The psychological type of the analyst and its relation to analytical practice. Journal of Analytical Psychology 23(3): 211–225.

Fordham M (1972) Note on *Psychological Types*. Journal of Analytical Psychology 17(2): 111–115.

Giegerich W (1977) On the neurosis of psychology or the third of the two. Spring: An Annual of Archetypal Psychology and Jungian Thought: 153–174.

Giegerich W (1998) The Soul's Logical Life: Towards a Rigorous Notion of Psychology. Frankfurt am Main: Peter Lang.

Groesbeck CL (1978) *Psychological Types* in the analysis of the transference. Journal of Analytical Psychology 23(1): 23–53.

Hillman J (1980) Egalitarian Typologies Versus the Perception of the Unique. Eranos Lectures 4. Dallas: Spring Publications.

Hillman J (1992) Revisioning Psychology. New York: HarperCollins.

Holt D (1987) 'Witness in theatre and behaviour'. In Hawkwood Papers 1979 to 1986. Oxford: privately printed.

Holt D (1998) 'Transference solicitation'. In Psyche in the Operating Theatre. Oxford: privately printed.

James W (1961) 'Report on Mrs Piper's Hodgson-Control'. In Murphy G, Ballou R (eds), William James on Psychical Research. London: Chatto and Windus.

Jung CG (1954) The Practice of Psychotherapy. Collected Works Volume 16. London: Routledge and Kegan Paul.

Jung CG (1962) The Archetypes and the Collective Unconscious. Collected Works Volume 9i. London: Routledge and Kegan Paul.

Jung CG (1963) Memories, Dreams, Reflections. Recorded and edited by Aniela Jaffe. New York: Pantheon Books.

Jung CG (1964) The Development of Personality. Collected Works Volume 17. London: Routledge and Kegan Paul.

Jung CG (1976) Psychological Types. Collected Works Volume 6. London: Routledge and Kegan Paul.

Jung CG (1977a) The Structure and Dynamics of the Psyche. Collected Works Volume 8. London: Routledge and Kegan Paul.

Jung CG (1977b) The Symbolic Life. Collected Works Volume 18. London: Routledge and Kegan Paul.

Jung CG (1990) Analytical Psychology: Notes of the Seminar Given in 1925, edited by McQuire W. London: Routledge.

Phillips A (1995) 'The story of the mind'. In Corrigan EG, Gordon PE (eds), The Mind Object: Precocity and Pathology of Self-Sufficiency. London: Karnac Books.

Roustang F (1958) Dire Mastery: Discipleship from Freud to Lacan. Baltimore: The Johns Hopkins University Press.

Shamdasani S (2003) Jung and the Making of Modern Psychology: The Dream of a Science. Cambridge: Cambridge University Press.

INDEX